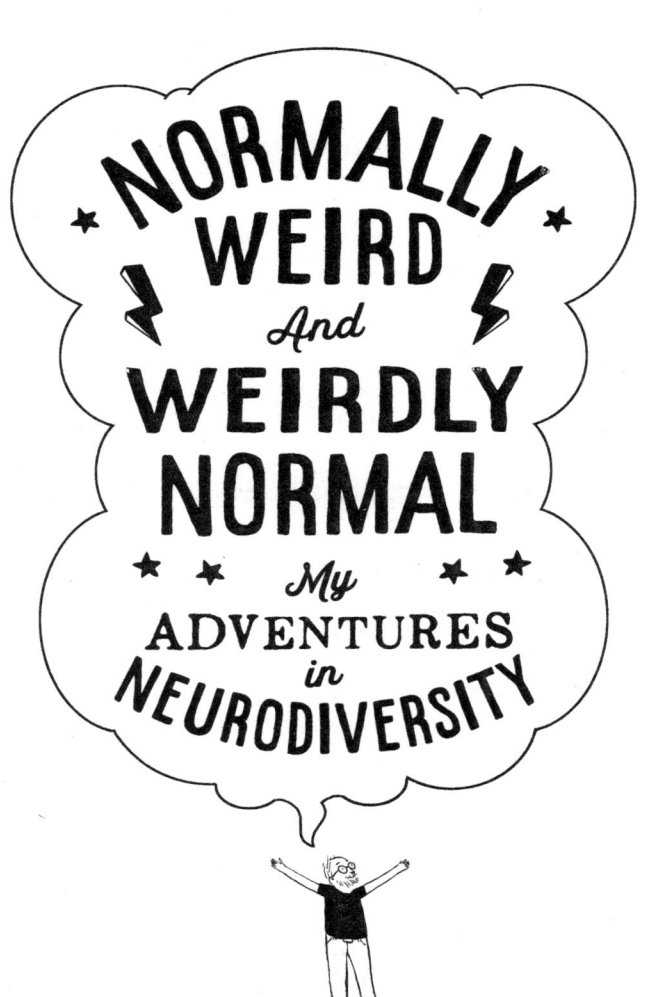

ABOUT THE AUTHOR

Robin Ince is a comedian, actor and writer. *The Guardian* once declared him a 'becardiganed polymath', which seems about right. He is the author of several acclaimed books, including *The Importance of Being Interested* and *I'm a Joke and So Are You*. With Professor Brian Cox, he created and presents the award-winning BBC Radio 4 show *The Infinite Monkey Cage*, which ranks among the most popular science podcasts worldwide. He also won *Celebrity Mastermind* but forgot that calcium was the dominant element of chalk. After being diagnosed with ADHD at the age of fifty-two, he finally has an excuse.

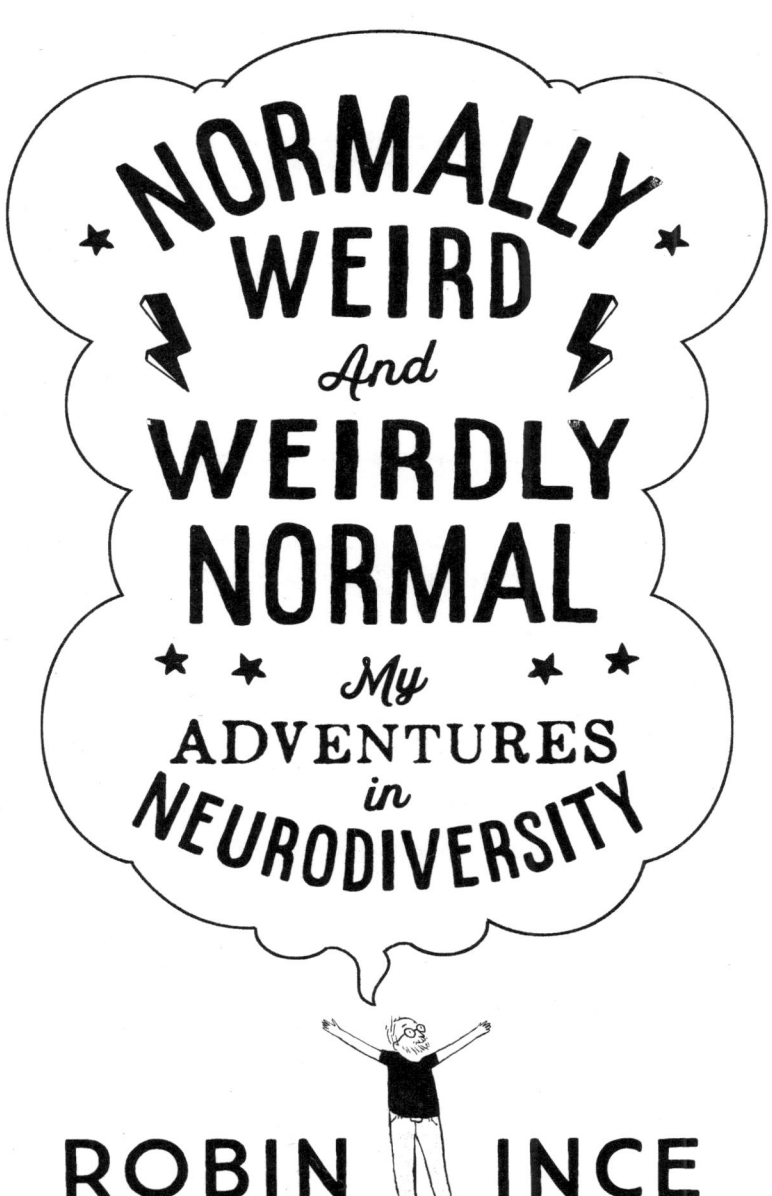

NORMALLY WEIRD And WEIRDLY NORMAL

My ADVENTURES in NEURODIVERSITY

ROBIN INCE

MACMILLAN

First published 2025 by Macmillan
an imprint of Pan Macmillan
The Smithson, 6 Briset Street, London EC1M 5NR
EU representative: Macmillan Publishers Ireland Ltd, 1st Floor,
The Liffey Trust Centre, 117–126 Sheriff Street Upper,
Dublin 1, D01 YC43
Associated companies throughout the world
www.panmacmillan.com

ISBN 978-1-0350-3692-9 HB
ISBN 978-1-0350-3693-6 TPB

Copyright © Robin Ince 2025

The right of Robin Ince to be identified as the
author of this work has been asserted by him in accordance
with the Copyright, Designs and Patents Act 1988.

All rights reserved. No part of this publication may be reproduced,
stored in a retrieval system, or transmitted, in any form, or by any means
(electronic, mechanical, photocopying, recording or otherwise)
without the prior written permission of the publisher.

Pan Macmillan does not have any control over, or any responsibility for,
any author or third-party websites referred to in or on this book.

1 3 5 7 9 8 6 4 2

A CIP catalogue record for this book is available from the British Library.

Chapter illustrations © Mecob 2025

Illustration on p.86 © Joanna Neary 2024

Typeset in Charter ITC Std by Palimpsest Book Production Ltd, Falkirk, Stirlingshire
Printed and bound by CPI Group (UK) Ltd, Croydon, CR0 4YY

This book is sold subject to the condition that it shall not, by way of
trade or otherwise, be lent, hired out, or otherwise circulated without
the publisher's prior consent in any form of binding or cover other than
that in which it is published and without a similar condition including
this condition being imposed on the subsequent purchaser.

Visit **www.panmacmillan.com** to read more about all our books
and to buy them. You will also find features, author interviews and
news of any author events, and you can sign up for e-newsletters
so that you're always first to hear about our new releases.

This book is dedicated to:

Ed, my friend of forty years.
'Remember Leningrad.'

Jamie and Lion, whose words
*'I think it might be worth exploring
the neurodivergent model a bit'* set me
on a new and far happier path.

And the SOLD charity shop in Shoreham.
Not only the most wondrous Aladdin's cave,
but also a place where people with learning
differences are truly shown their worth
and potential.

CONTENTS

A Brief Note   ix

INTRODUCTION – BUT YOU ARE WEIRD   1

1. CRASH!   25

2. WEIRDO or WHEN DID YOU REALIZE YOU WERE ODD?   53

3. FRIENDSHIP   77

4. THE CONVERSATION   91

5. WORK (IS A FOUR-LETTER WORD)   103

6. HOARDING, COLLECTING AND OBSESSIONS   129

7. POLITICS AND KINDNESS   151

8. LOVE AND OTHER CATASTROPHES   165

9. COUCH or HOW I MET ME   185

10. REVELATION or THANK YOU UNMASKED MAN   199

11. DIAGNOSIS – I DID, WHAT ABOUT YOU?   211

12. MADDER WHEN SANE   229

AFTERWORD   247

Endnotes   251

Index   259

A BRIEF NOTE

Throughout this book, you will find many people referred to by their first name only.

My research has consisted of many direct interviews but has also drawn on people's reaction to questions I've posed on social media. Although all of those I engaged with on social media were fully aware their input may well be used in this book, I decided that I would not use their full names because, though society is hopefully becoming less judgemental about people's mental health, there is still a way to go and not everyone wants their work colleagues etc. to know their inner workings.

I would also like to make it clear that, though this book may veer towards appealing to those who are defined as neurodivergent, I think being human is weird from the outset. However neurotypical you may be, you are still a weirdo to me, and I mean that as a compliment.

INTRODUCTION – BUT YOU ARE WEIRD

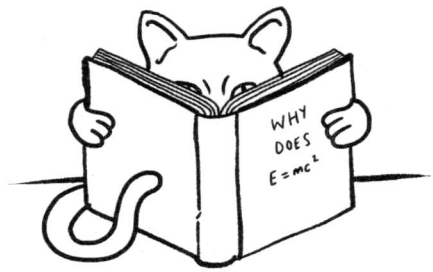

I am not going to beat around the bush.

I am weird.

I've always known I was weird, but if I was in any doubt, then my wife has often reminded me by saying, 'Why do you always say such weird things?' as yet another bemused person walks away from me at a party.

She is not alone. I am very good at engendering quizzical looks. My long-time touring and podcast partner, Professor Brian Cox, has a habit of saying, 'You know that no one knows what you're talking about?' But this is not entirely true. Some people know exactly what I'm talking about, and it turns out there are more of them than you might imagine. Though there are some who walk away at gatherings, there are others who I make an instant lifelong connection with. You might be one of them and, if not, hopefully you will be by the end of this book.

But before we break down our weirds, let's address the elephant in the room: however normal you think you are, you are weird.

For instance, you are reading words. Does your cat read books? Does your hamster do crosswords? Does your dog worry that its new collar doesn't go with its ears? And while we are on that topic, why does your dog insist on having sex with another dog so indiscreetly, going for it in the park in broad daylight in front of the Salvation Army band?

Even if you do not consider yourself a weird human, your weirdness is inescapable because you are a human, and in the natural order of things, to be human is to be quite odd.

You have inner thoughts. They help you know you are alive. You experience shame. You use complex language. You say things you don't mean. You want to be in charge, but there are things that are out of your hands. You cannot argue yourself out of an upset stomach or truly fake a smile or stop yourself blushing. You cannot control who you fall in love with, and you can't always persuade them to fall in love with you back. You are aware that others may be judging you, even though you can't hear them say a thing. You know that one day you will die and the world will continue without you. That is a lot to take on.

So however normal you think you are, always remember you are weird.

By our current understanding, beyond being one of the rare living things to inhabit the universe, it is your thoughts that are your greatest oddity. We are more than one thing. There is an inside us and an outside us. There is who we present ourselves as being and who we believe ourselves to be. We often spend much, if not all, of our time concealing what our real thoughts are, and it is this elaborate charade that is the cause of many problems.

As a therapist once told me, the problem with being human is that we judge everyone else from their exterior and ourselves from the interior. Most of the time, you don't know what is going on in my mind and I don't know what is going on in yours, and from this basic state of being grow many fears – a fear of honesty and a fear of expression – as well as many presumptions about how minds should work, the presumptions of what it is to be normal.

If someone breaks the silence by asking, 'What are you thinking?' how often do you reply honestly? The larger a society becomes, the more interactions there may be, the greater the number of rules and the greater the number of deceptions. We deceive other people, and we deceive ourselves. We judge ourselves by a standard which it might turn out no one else is meeting.

The unbearable rules of being normal

We have rules that apply to business, sex, gender, religious belief, love, domesticity, morality, politics, and rules that direct attitudes to people who are not considered to be inside the group or behaving as the group should. Those who do not obey the rules are seen as threats or failures or impositions or, sometimes, worthy of execution.

Some societies see no problem with same-sex relationships, while others believe such love should be punished by death. Some societies have two genders, while others recognize more, such as the hijra and sekrata. Some people believe it is the 'natural law' for men to dominate, while others have done a bit more reading. Some people don't believe that there are gods in the sky, while others demand that those who question their god must be stoned to death. Often, once the powerful in a society have sanctioned the rules, those rules become immutable law, and those who question those laws are outliers and outlaws.

The playwright and comedian Francesca Martinez called her memoir of growing up *What the F*** Is Normal?* She defines herself as 'wobbly', which is how she refers to her cerebral palsy. She was judged by many to have almost no potential as a child. Though cerebral palsy is related to movement, many people assume all those with cerebral palsy also have issues with their minds. Francesca's parents fought for her rights. She has been a successful actor and comedian and is now an award-winning playwright, but as a child, the 'normal' presumptions were that she should just have been left in the corner.

NORMALLY WEIRD AND WEIRDLY NORMAL

The autistic naturalist Dara McAnulty was similarly written off, but by sixteen years old, he had written an award-winning book, *Diary of a Young Naturalist* (I recommend it to you all), and has gone on to study at Cambridge University.

They are just two examples of why it is important to look beyond what is considered 'normal'. If we just accept the rules, we can dash so much potential on the rocks. There are people everywhere who have massive potential but have been written off because of what are considered their unsurmountable mental or physical disabilities, their 'quirks', when all we are really talking about is their difference from the 'norm'.

We might think of 'normal' as the mean average of how humans behave, but it is not even that, as behaviour that falls too far from expectations is entirely ignored when mapping the averages and creating the rules. And so it seems to me that, often, normal is just about creating people who cause the least inconvenience to society and appear to be the most similar in shape and colour to those with the most power.

One of the arrogances of many is that they believe that the way they see the world is the correct and utterly objective way of seeing the world. Too many people want to insist that they are right and you are wrong. No one has access to some sort of objective reality. This doesn't mean there aren't ideas that are useful for your survival, and it doesn't mean all opinions are equally valid.

Whatever our differences in beliefs about deities or physics, if you and I jump off a hundred-storey building at the same time, it is likely we will end up being raspberry jam at pretty much the same moment. Our physical interaction with the world around us, whether to extreme heat, high speed, starvation or arrows, will be pretty much the same (I try to avoid all four). But our inner life, our thoughts and emotional reactions to the world, can be very different. Our expectations of the world are one of the things that make our world what it is, and our expectations are shaped by our experience.

INTRODUCTION – BUT YOU ARE WEIRD

This is not just about emotional reactions. It can be that we have genuinely different sensory experiences due to the culture and environment around us. An example often drawn upon is that of the Himba tribe of Namibia. They do not see a difference between blue and green, but can place shades of green into far more categories than Europeans. Their language has far more names for shades of green, and with that comes a far greater ability to perceive different greens.

In the film world, research into on-screen gender imbalance shows that if a woman talks as much as a man in a scene, she is considered to have had far more screen time; and if one third of characters in a scene are women, then the audience judge it as being over half.

The screenwriter and director Alice Lowe told me that you are only allowed one weird. As a straight, white, middle-class male, my weird could be that I am 'a little weird'. She explained that being a woman is her weird already, in far too many people's eyes. The fact that she then wrote a screenplay about a pregnant woman being told by the embryo inside her to murder certain men is seen as just too darn weird.*

I have seen such treatment dished out to many female friends in the arts, those who have dared to express a creativity that goes beyond what is deemed the right and proper way for women to create and perform. We still live in a world where someone can confidently say, 'Women just aren't funny,' as if that person's inability to find women funny is an inalienable truth that must be held by all others and that those laughing are only doing so because they are 'politically correct' or some other such jazz. Some even go as far as to create evolutionary theories of why women have not developed to be funny. This has nothing to do with hard science and, again, much to do with society's expectations.

---

* That film is *Prevenge* and I recommend it. You'll really cheer when that man is stabbed in the genitals.

NORMALLY WEIRD AND WEIRDLY NORMAL

I once witnessed an incident in a bookshop in Belper. An already outraged man in red trousers walked in, took a brief glance at the fiction, most of which happened to be written by women, and loudly exclaimed, 'I see you don't stock any books for middle-aged white men!' As a middle-aged white man, he could not imagine that the books of Margaret Atwood, Edna O'Brien, Emily Brontë, Toni Morrison could offer anything for him because they would be too infiltrated with lady-ness; he might be fearful that feminine words could make him womanly and he would start wearing an indigo skirt rather than his manly red trousers.

You might think that this is a bit tangential, but that may happen every now and again in a book about neurodivergence written by someone diagnosed with attention deficit hyperactivity disorder (ADHD). (Did I mention I was ADHD, sorry if I forgot, I do get easily distracted, but there's plenty of time for that.) Personally, I think it is a good starting point for mulling over how easily some people dismiss the reality of other people's minds and how they can slip into the belief that 'if you don't think like me then you have something wrong because I am most definitely normal'.

'Normal' is relative. Perhaps, rather than thinking of people being 'abnormal' or 'weird', we should just acknowledge that their way of being is rarer. 'Normal' certainly does not mean being innately right or good. But changing attitudes about what is generally accepted as normal can be a slow and protracted process, facing much resistance, especially from those who profit by keeping the system as it is.

This book is about our mental life, about judgement predominantly based on thoughts rather than appearance. It makes people feel ill at ease, scared, when seemingly weird thoughts spring from people that look like them. Who knows, maybe it's catching and they could become weird next. Is being overly tangential, wildly curious and deeply passionate about things that may be highly esoteric catching? I hope so!

But perhaps things are changing as many people begin to find the

INTRODUCTION - BUT YOU ARE WEIRD

corridors of normality too narrow. They may have behaved all their lives as if all was okay and they may have been obedient to the rules, but often at a great mental cost to themselves. Some have disguised their 'abnormality' for the whole of their unhappy lives, and others may have snapped. Some have destroyed themselves, some have lashed out and destroyed others due to the stresses of trying to maintain their illusion. Some people may have visibly not fitted in from the outset and borne the brunt of other people's judgement and disdain.

What has become known as neurodivergence can be so difficult for some to mask, so difficult to match with the rules of being 'normal', that such people have become marginalized, increasing their trauma and generating further negative thoughts about themselves.

I believe that there are far more unhappy and anxious people in the world than is necessary (whatever the necessary number for unhappiness is) and that it is the rules we live by that are not fit for purpose. Many of us have been secretive for too long about our struggles to toe the line with these rules. The spectrum of ways that our brains perceive and interpret the world clashes with the rules, rules that state there is an objectively correct way of behaving and perceiving. If you don't follow the rules and interact correctly, then you are admonished, shamed, mocked or excluded.

So perhaps it is time to change the rules, to change our perceptions of what it is to be normal, to broaden our understanding of the varieties of ways people think, and to challenge whether there is such a thing as normal at all. This is undoubtedly an exciting time, greatly illuminated by the concept of neurodiversity.

Neurodiversity

The word 'neurodiversity' was coined by academic and activist Judy Singer in 1997. She explained that '"Neuro" was a reference to the rise of neuroscience. "Diversity" is a political term; it originated with the black American civil rights movement. "Biodiversity" is really a political term, too. As a word, "neurodiversity" describes the whole of humanity. But the neurodiversity *movement* is a political movement for people who want their human rights.'[1]

It is important to understand then that, while not everyone is neurodivergent, we are all neurodiverse. Neurodiversity is a way to understand the variety of ways human minds behave and react in, and to, the world. It challenges the simplicity of saying there are only two positions – you are either mentally well or mentally ill, your brain is either working 'right' or working 'wrong'. If it is not working 'correctly', you must disguise it, as people would prefer that rather than be presented with any flamboyant revelations. The neurodivergent throws down a gauntlet to such a single-minded view of the world.

The neurodiversity movement was initially attached to autism or autism spectrum disorder (ASD), and over the years there has been a great change in the understanding of what it is to be autistic. Neurodivergence now also includes ADHD, dyspraxia and dyslexia.

To be neurodivergent is to have a mind that finds a myriad of challenges in engaging with the world as it has been constructed. The neurodiversity movement challenges this construction and those who insist that this is the only way. It turns the pressure away from the neurodivergent to meekly obey the rules. It challenges the presumption that any failure to engage correctly with the world is *your* failure, and instead says, 'Maybe there has been a severe lack of imagination and empathy in the way society has been structured and rules made.'

The demand for a world where one size fits all has already been challenged by picking apart the notion that 'the average human' was deemed to be the one with the Y chromosome. Women, if they were a concern at all in scientific, medical and technical research, were a peripheral issue unless the focus was on how their wombs made them mad during the hysteria boom years.

INTRODUCTION – BUT YOU ARE WEIRD

During the hysteria age of the mid- to late nineteenth century, where 'hysterical' women would be put on display like a twisted talent show, it was decided men could also have hysteria, but only if they had flabby testicles. I think it might have been the testicle-squeezing flabbiness-check that might have brought on the hysteria.

Hopefully, the twenty-first century will be the century where such ideas are finally disposed of, but there are many with wealth and power who continue to fight for a return to the systems that have treated them so well.

Masking

Masking plays an important part in the understanding of the problems that can come from trying to adhere to social rules, from anxiety and from having a neurodivergent state of mind. I have only recently come to realize that I have been masking my whole life, pretending and hiding, just as I was expected to do.

For example, for three decades my wife had no idea that, at pretty much any given moment during that time, I was constantly wracked by anxiety. My mind was a Rolodex of persistent worries, only occasionally blotted out by being on stage or getting truly lost in a book. If I wasn't worrying about what I had already done wrong, I was worrying about what I was about to do wrong.

There is a habit among those paid to type up their opinions and among those who do it for free on social media to say 'it was never like this in the olden days' with all this masking, mental health issues and non-binary young people, dismissing such things as being something our grandfathers and grandmothers would never have bothered with in the war or as they buried their fifth child in a pauper's grave. They 'just got on with it'. And sometimes this may have been true, but often it was not. It does them a disservice to suggest that they didn't have finely tuned human minds too, that they weren't sensitive to fears, pains, stress and anxiety about how they fitted in and survived in the world. One autistic TikToker responded to this cynicism with the simple response, 'Europeans didn't know Everest existed until 1852, but I'm pretty sure it was there before that.'

I believe more people are aware that what we experience of someone is not necessarily what is going on inside their heads, but many are not aware just how extreme the disparity might be. A most tragic example is the shock we might feel when someone who appeared to us to be the happy-go-lucky life and soul of the party takes their own life. We like to imagine that there would have been clear signs of depression and that they would have been expressed. We punish ourselves for not noticing when there might have been nothing to see.

Women have often had to mask their characters and identities to fit in with wide-ranging social restrictions such as not sitting in the cigar room and drinking brandy, or alone in a pub not wanting attention, or knowing more than a man about politics or fluid dynamics. LGBT people have had to hide both their love and desire. And the more I researched this book, the more I discovered just how many people have to mask in so many different parts of their lives. And so, to 'fit in' and get on in life, to not stand out, to not be shunned, to not be mocked, and even to not be attacked or killed, people have to mask who they really are on more than one level.

'Masking' is the process of concealing the reality of your experience. It is forcing yourself to don the uncomfortable disguise of someone who says, 'Oh yes, it is all okay. I am not anxious/depressed/suicidal/unable to concentrate on a word you're saying/not interested, etc.' It is making the conversation you think you are meant to be making, while inside you are screaming, 'I am so BORED! And I am being so BORING! What on earth am I talking about?' It is staying quiet so that you don't 'rock the boat', even if the boat-rocking may lead to better results and empty the bilge tank. (I have never tried a flooded-boat analogy before, so I hope that worked for any yacht-racers or pleasure-boaters.)

INTRODUCTION - BUT YOU ARE WEIRD

You might be in a room where everyone is masking and pretending they are not frustrated and exhausted (you probably are in such a room, all the time) but, as no one has loosened the elastic that keeps the disguise in place, you would never know, and neither would they.

For me, this is one of the joys of performing stand-up comedy, that you can let out the hidden voice inside you and the people watching can come to realize they are not alone. I have always been lucky enough to have had a space where I can express myself freely, or as freely as my mind and my own fear will allow me.

And now all about me, me, me . . .

This book exists because of the enormous change in my happiness about being alive.

A stranger was generous enough to contact me because they were concerned that I didn't realize what was going on in my own head. When I found out about my neurodivergence, there was an elated silence. Yet it was also a silence so full of thoughts, so full of relief, so full of revelations and understanding, that the cacophony went beyond incessant and into silence. There was so much to hear that I could hear nothing. I found myself, but I seemed lost for words.

After a lengthy conversation, the stranger had concluded that I had a mind that could be classified as 'neurodivergent', specifically ADHD. Understanding myself as being ADHD was so immense, and it has changed me so much. I think for anyone who has not experienced this, who finds that they sit reasonably comfortably within their mind, this might be hard to understand, and it can be easy to dismiss, and so I hope this book goes some way to showing how life-changing such a discovery was for me and can be for so many.

I had a totally new understanding of how I worked and who I was. I suddenly experienced so many feelings and saw so many new possibilities. These feelings could not be captured in a single sentence. Lucky really, or this would be a very short book.

It was a Eureka! moment without me feeling the need to run naked and dripping through the streets shouting about it. Which was also fortunate, because it would have been a pity if a new joy about my sanity led to me being put in an insane asylum for my sodden nudity.

I felt I was a different human being. Or rather, I was exactly the same human being as I always was, but now I had a new instruction manual that explained how my mind worked. Though I am very bad at reading assembly manuals and will improvise after the second instruction to slot A into B before folding over into C (one of the reasons that much of the furniture in my house is haunted with jeopardy), the existence of a manual was succour in itself. Also, I now had a tangible reason for my asymmetrical sofa beds.

Decades of self-loathing, suicidal thoughts, frustration, anxiety, and a persistent critical voice that could lavish failure over any possible success, thinned and eventually faded.

Suddenly, everything made sense.

Well, not *everything*. I still have trouble with wave particle duality and Kant's *Critique of Pure Reason*, and David Lynch's *Mulholland Drive* remains enigmatic. The problems of the laws of the universe and of experimental cinema remained, but the problems of being me were greatly reduced. I realize this is not a rare story. And this book will not just be my story. Understanding me more was a very useful tool for starting to understand other people more. This book has evolved from simply having the tool of a new prism to interrogate the world with.

For most of my life, I don't think I would have accepted that I was neurodivergent. I was just perpetually anxious about the screaming banshees in my head telling me I was rubbish and a failure and had let everyone down, while spending my downtime daydreaming about hanging under a bridge. It's just a way of life, isn't it? What it

INTRODUCTION - BUT YOU ARE WEIRD

is to be human? Like all those wonderfully miserable Scandinavian films I watched about the lost and the lonely and those poets I read who had retreated into constant pessimism. Surely that was an easier and even more admirable existence than striving for happiness.

What surprises me now is that I couldn't see it before and that I felt it would be wrong to try to improve my situation. Everything I now know about my mind and its behaviour, or 'me' as I call it, was there all the time. It wasn't as if I didn't know about neurodivergence. I had even written about it and talked about it on stage, but always referring to it in the context of other people and not myself.

Had I been in denial? What is it that gives us the vision to diagnose other people and fail to see things in ourselves? After my stand-up shows, people would often come up to me and say, 'I'm neurodivergent, good to know you are too.' Sometimes they would suggest I was on the autistic spectrum, sometimes that I was ADHD, and sometimes they would even say that I was displaying aspects of being bipolar. I would always tell them it was just my stage persona and no more. I was avoiding the obvious, which was that my stage self was the truest exhibition of what was going on at all times in my waking mind.

On stage has always been where I have felt freest and the most in control, despite it also being where I appear at my most chaotic. It is where I have been able to open my mind to others and let it run as wild as my imagination would take it, while always being confined by the limitations of a nagging critical voice. Performance has helped me to work out how to stop performing during the rest of my life, making the disparity between who I am on stage and who I am off it almost non-existent.

'I had been surrounded by it and yet hadn't realized I had it myself'[2]

My failure to see what was right behind my nose all that time is a common phenomenon. Sarah Hendrickx had been working exclusively in the field of autism diagnosis for five years before she realized she herself was on the autistic spectrum. In *Women and Girls with Autism Spectrum Disorder*, she writes, 'It seems ludicrous even to me that someone so immersed in both the theory and practice of autism could not spot it in herself.' She even wrote a book with her autistic husband about what it was like to be a neurotypical person in a relationship with someone autistic. Thinking about how she was able to understand her husband, when so many other neurotypical people didn't, became a major factor on the way to understanding herself.

She realized that her outward presentation was 'deliberately and extremely well-constructed'. Her failure to see herself as she was, despite her expertise, was partly because she had been trained in a world where autism has been seen as being a particularly male condition and the tests for it have been very skewed to male autistic behaviour, while some scientists have written about how 'specific aspects of autistic neuroanatomy may also be extremes of typical male neuroanatomy'.[3] She was also coping well with life, another impediment to diagnosis for many neurodivergent people, because if you are coping, few people are that interested in you. Some people can create the illusion of keeping themselves together while unravelling for a lifetime.

Hendrickx also writes about the different standards she had for herself. There were many neurodivergent people in her family, and she never considered them or any of the autistic people she worked with to be inadequate; yet, for her, the idea of being different made her 'a less than perfectly acceptable person', something I can strongly identify with from my past.

INTRODUCTION - BUT YOU ARE WEIRD

Many of us have two sets of standards: one for those we know and love, and a totally different set of unreachable standards for ourselves. What we happily accept in others, we see as terrible failings in ourselves. The failure to 'fit in', whether inwardly or outwardly, is your terrible failure.

Try harder

For many years, I played the part of who I thought I should have been pretty well, while on the inside, I was picking myself apart and finding abject failure in any success.

It is surprisingly easy to be deeply unhappy and for no one to know it. I travelled through life with someone else alongside me. They thought I was pathetic and embarrassing and wouldn't hesitate to tell me at every opportunity. There was a persistent sneering heckler living with me. The one who knew the truth. After I finished a gig I would leave any hecklers behind in the comedy club, but the real heckler came with me, slept with me, woke with me, and every step I took, he took too.

I hope it doesn't sound crass, but this self-hating is the model of an abusive relationship. You are living with someone who is constantly belittling you and saying you don't deserve anything better. Tragically, this sort of internal relationship centred on worthlessness can often lead to people becoming trapped in relationships with other people who do exactly the same to them. Those who frequently judge themselves harshly are at an increased risk of getting into relationships where they are controlled and/or abused, because inside they feel that they deserve no better.

Who else would want this useless specimen? How much easier it is to psychologically abuse someone who is already psychologically abusing themselves. Many of those I talked to have found themselves relentless victims of bullying and systemic abuse. I am glad to say that many have escaped when they came to know themselves.

NORMALLY WEIRD AND WEIRDLY NORMAL

This is true in the workplace too, where employers feel empowered by an atmosphere that allows them to say, 'You are lucky to have a job with us,' and is why the status quo may well be resistant to new paradigms of behaviour and understanding. Why would those controlling society want to change it, when anxiety and low self-esteem are so useful for manipulation?

The expected normal

My friend Jo has experienced that internal and external abuse. I may not see her for years, but when we see each other, our friendship carries on just the same as the last time we met, and we pick up wherever the last conversation ended. Both of us have had significant changes in our life since we first met and both of us are far more knowledgeable now about how we diverge from the expected 'normal'.

I first saw Jo when she was tap-dancing at a late-night cabaret event in 2006. I love watching tap-dancing. I would love to be a tap-dancer, and I dream of being Gene Kelly. I used to dance around our living room imagining I was Fred Astaire after watching *Top Hat*, but really, I was whirling like a Tasmanian devil.* Sadly, I lack syncopated feet. To be honest, I lack syncopated everything.

As I watched Jo, I was struck by one of my *brilliant* ideas. Her tap-dancing would be the perfect accompaniment to the readings from the Mills and Boon books I was performing dramatic readings from on a nightly basis. It would particularly enhance the confrontation scene between the passionate, but frustrated, sheep farmer and the ingénue shearer from the big city in the final chapter of *Rash Intruder* – 'Autocratic, short-tempered and demanding was how Tamar summed up her new boss, trouble-shooter Dagan Carmichael. He was also incredibly attractive . . .'[4]

---

* 'Looney Tunes', not your natural history variety.

INTRODUCTION – BUT YOU ARE WEIRD

After the show, I bounded up to Jo, all smiles and creative excitement and blurted out, 'Your dancing was great. I am doing a show where I read out from 1970s romantic fiction about antipodean rural pursuits and lighthouse keepers, as well as novels about giant killer crab invasions, and I think your tap dancing would add a whole new dimension to the stories of dreamy looks over the ram-castrating shears and pincer severings.'

We look back now and realize that this is apparently not a standard neurotypical opening gambit.

The next day, she was on stage with me, and that was the beginning of a beautiful friendship forged through dance and budget romantic fiction. I am surprised that such a scenario hasn't been used more often in the movies (I don't know why my screenplays keep being rejected).

It is an example of the shortcuts that are typical of neurodivergent relationships, of just getting straight to the point and not disguising any excitable emotions. I have never understood all the hidden games of social conversations, the questions that are frequently asked without any real interest and with very little interest given in the replies, a dull role-playing of necessary reality. How many of us teach ourselves the rules and then miss the opportunity for exploring far more fascinating tangents.

Having seen little of each other for over a decade, I met Jo at a bookshop, my place of exuberant delight, and I straight away took to recommending books, no outback sheep-dip love stories this time. I told Jo that she must read Kirsty Loehr's *A Short History of Queer Women*, a book I adored because it is fascinating and written as if you are in a pub with a friend who is two beers in and excitedly telling you about all the latest things they've found out about the world.

It is said that the poet Sappho invented the Lesbian somewhere between c.620 and 570 BCE. Men had been screwing each other for a while back then. We know this is true because it had been written about (by men), sung about (by men) and encouraged (by women repulsed by men).[5]

Jo beamingly bought a copy.

It was only when we were in the pub next door that I discovered I had missed the news that Jo had come out since we last met.

Uh oh.

Had it sounded like I was being a patronizing, middle-aged man and that I was recommending Kirsty's book like an overcompensating liberal idiot? A terrible pillar of the patriarchy? 'Hey Jo, just so you know, I am pretty cool about you being a lesbian, actually I read lesbian books too, reckon you should read this book, will give you a good sense of your history . . .' Once, I would have panicked and my berating inner monologue would have bellowed admonishment; but now, that heckler in my head was powerless. Those multiple layers of paranoia had been stripped away. And Jo, after years of concealment, can now be happily open about her sexuality and her neurodivergence.

It may seem surprising, but if you saw us chatting together, we would look just as we did when we first met, and yet inside, both of us are radically different. Jo is one of the many examples of people in my life with whom I instantly clicked, perhaps because in some subconscious way we were drawn together by the things we didn't understand about ourselves and each other.

I think perhaps now I might even have less anxiety than the average person, and while I can't promise to cure you, later in the book I will give it a damn good try. (I should probably have put this big promise even earlier in the book to snare the casual browser. I'll make up for it now.)

I WILL CURE YOU OF YOUR ANXIETY.*

---

* Terms and conditions apply.

INTRODUCTION – BUT YOU ARE WEIRD

I am armed with a new confidence and a new happiness, and this is perhaps why I can walk unafraid into the bear pit of cynics and nay-sayers with the writing of this book. Like every major change in our society, in understanding of ourselves, there is resistance from those who demand that we go back to the good ole days where no one was happy and everyone died young, those who are dismissive of this all being the latest fad, a psychological version of fidget spinners or twerking. If it is the latest fad, then this is a rare moment where I may be fashionable.

One of the highest profile documentaries about ADHD on British television was about the dangers of ADHD being over-diagnosed. This fitted very nicely into the cynic's narrative of 'most of you are making all this up for attention' or 'get over yourselves, you're just not strong enough for the real world'.

A more responsible documentary might have focused on a far more pressing issue – not that some people may be being misdiagnosed (a real possibility) but that thousands are waiting years for a diagnosis at all. As so often, our short-term save-money approach is costing far more in the long term as people battle alone with their mental health.

But I have been cynical too. As some of my closest friends were getting diagnosed, I would think, *But all this melancholy and confusion and babbling of voices is just being a human, isn't it? What's the fuss?* I was deflecting. I am not sure if this was denial or some innate 'you've got to keep calm and carry on – it is the British way' type of thinking. But I've come to realize that, for many, 'keep calm and carry on' is actually 'conceal your despair and stumble on'.

I think I was lucky. I did not seek a diagnosis; one came to me. And then another one after that, and this is all part of the story you are about to read.

NORMALLY WEIRD AND WEIRDLY NORMAL

Why a book?

The older I have become, the more important it has become for me to have a reason to write and perform. When I was an aspirational kid, I only wanted to be an author, and then I wanted to be a comedian. It was as I met middle age that I found what satisfied me most. I love showing off and I love showing off for a purpose even more.

In 2023, I made a radio series called *Reality Tunnel* about the outside and inside of our heads, predominantly using my own head as the default model. I received a lot of feedback after the broadcast. One of my favourite comments was from a 67-year-old man. He said that he had lived his life believing his mind was the only one that contained the 'weird' thoughts that were persistently being conjured up. After listening to my show, he realized he was not alone. He now knew that there may be plenty of other people with eccentric and absurd noises and rapid and random thoughts buzzing around inside their heads, and if there weren't plenty, then at least there were two. A parent once told me that, after hearing me fizz my way through a gig, her daughter had turned to her and said, 'Mum, that's what my head sounds like.'

As I have become freer in the way I express myself publicly, I have met more and more people who have had their mind described as being similar, and I have found it exciting to communicate and connect with such people.

In Lowestoft, a couple approached me, one of them tearful, and his partner said, 'He is going through diagnosis now and it is the first time he has publicly seen something like his brain on display.' In a world of conformity, where difference can easily be seen as a threat and people strike first when they feel threatened, it's common to feel isolated and lost.

So I am writing this book because I do not believe there is such a thing as a normal human being, but that there are normal ways we

INTRODUCTION – BUT YOU ARE WEIRD

are expected to behave and think; and that many people are terrified of breaking those social norms and many go along with them, even though they don't really know why the norms are there. Living in a world that expects us to obey such a rigid set of rules ultimately deprives us of a far more interesting place to live. Of innovation and creativity, of love and friendships.

The greater the disparity between how we show ourselves to the world and what we really experience in our heads, the greater our potential unhappiness. We grow tired and distressed from our own constant cognitive dissonance. I would like the world to be a place where someone doesn't get to be sixty-seven years old before they realize that they are 'not the only one'.

It is not good enough to say 'Well, if you are getting through your day and surviving in the world, that should be enough.' There is enough upset, anxiety and melancholy that is inescapable, so why suffer when it is not necessary? Suffering in silence is best left to masochist monks. If a happier life can be made, then we should work hard to make sure it is available to as many people as possible.

The avant-garde composer and mushroom forager John Cage was once asked by the artist Robert Rauschenberg if there was too much suffering in the world. He replied that he thought there was just the right amount, a typically Zen reply. I would like to disagree with Cage, and perhaps the Buddha on this. I think there is too much suffering, and even if there is the right amount, then it is not evenly distributed.

On terminology

I currently appear to have an ADHD mind, but in the future that wording may change, even if my mind's behaviour does not. I believe that if the world can move forward, then psychological labelling, perhaps even the need for medication, will become less necessary. Some of the medicalized will become normalized.

NORMALLY WEIRD AND WEIRDLY NORMAL

We are also increasingly seeing that many people on the autistic spectrum are also ADHD, and some are bipolar or dyslexic or dyspraxic too.

Biology and psychology are complicated. I think this is why some physicists I know balk at psychology in the same way some dismiss abstract art or experimental jazz funk. However complex a subatomic particle might appear as we look at the equations concerning quantum behaviour in our probabilistic universe, that seems easy to comprehend when compared to understanding living minds and their neural pathways.

The regimentation of a single label or a diagnosis does not really account for the complexity of how many things we can be. For those who energetically question this, perhaps ask yourself why this widening understanding of our neurodiversity is threatening or problematic for you? How much does the increase of others potential happiness make your life sadder or more problematic? Why does the greater variety of ways of reacting and interacting with the world unsettle us if those ways are benign?

So this book is not about the neurodivergent and the neurotypical. It is about lots and lots of minds, some labelled autistic, some labelled ADHD, some labelled neurotypical, some undiagnosed or undecided, but all human minds that demonstrate the magnificent variety of what can be, so long as we don't have to live in a world where it is believed that one way must fit all. The speed with which our society wants to make people 'weirdos' or outsiders means too much has been concealed for too long. As more people talk openly, more people in hiding can see themselves and come forth.

Henry David Thoreau famously wrote that most of us live 'lives of quiet desperation', and for some, there may be very tangible reasons for this; but for others, this life 'of quiet desperation' and the costs that come with it – the cost of concealing ourselves – is something I believe to be almost entirely unnecessary.

Walk into an art gallery or a science museum and wonder how

INTRODUCTION – BUT YOU ARE WEIRD

much emptier they would be if every mind had a uniform reaction to the world. Do we even need poetry in a world where everything is so sure and certain and nailed down? You wouldn't need a variety of music, we'd all just be at the same Foo Fighters gig, and one joke would be suitable and funny for everyone. It is precisely because of the variety of possible ways of being in the world that we are such a creative species. So until we can live in a society where people can be honest, we must consider how many Einsteins or William Blakes there may be keeping themselves and their creativity silent.

Just to remind you one more time, we are *all* weird. Complex language, inner monologues, the need to understand why we are here and how the universe began, cinnamon-scented plug-in air fresheners, shame, cuckoo clocks, Bikram yoga, scientology – however normal you may be, you are still a member of the weirdest species in the known universe.

How this book works

This is not a self-help book, but I hope it helps. It is not a science book, but I hope, where I can be accurate about the neuroscience and psychology, I have been accurate. This is not a pop-up book . . .

Err, that's it – it really isn't a pop-up book. Much as I love them, I am not a paper technologist, sorry.

A necessary footnote

Before we begin, I think it is important for me to note that I am aware that my experience and my battles with my neurodivergent head and the world have been made easier by my privilege. I see the intersectional view of the world as important. I know that race, sex, gender and class will all bring with them different experiences and different problems. I hope that this look at the inner world will at least create common ground from which we can open up conversations.

1. CRASH!

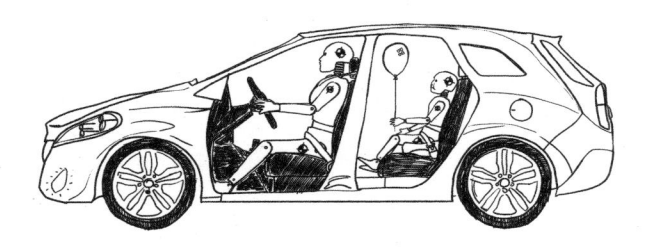

Why is my mind?

It is incredibly useful, but sadly rare, to know why you are as you are. Some people don't want to know. They plough forward in life and may only glance back occasionally, perhaps when they dig up the odd skeleton. I am still that five-year-old boy who constantly asks, 'But why? But why? But why?' I take very little for granted, especially when it comes to human behaviour, both mine and other people's. My head always needs to be thinking about something, and I have always spent a lot of time thinking about you (and about me).

How you and me have become who we are is a messy question of nature and nurture, but we can build up a set of clues and stories which might help plot a way through the jumble. In trying to understand why our minds can be so diverse in the ways they interact with the world, we need to consider our genetics, specific infant experiences (even such as premature birth), childhood experiences (loss, sudden change, poverty, abuse, war) and multiple other variables. We carry our experiences with us, from trust issues to post-traumatic stress disorder (PTSD). The events of our past are not left behind each New Year's Day as the bells toll; they come with us, even when we appear to have forgotten them. As unique individuals, we might experience the very same event in the same location, but it does not mean that we will be affected in the same way. Our experience of the same thing may be very different.

Some people may not be affected at all by an experience that was hugely impactful to someone else. One person might be rescued from a burning building and see it as little more than a good anecdote for when things are getting dull at a party. Others might go through the same event and develop PTSD, and as a result their lives might tumble into a spiral of fear, anxiety and despair.

It has been written that the human brain is the most complex thing in the known universe. That's perhaps why scientists like to use nematode worms to study how brains work, as the worms only have 302 cells in their nervous system, whereas humans have about 100 billion cells in their brains. Nevertheless, as relatively straightforward as they are, the nematode worm's nerve cells still make thousands of different connections, so even their simple minds are not so simple. The more pathways, the more possibilities. For worms, as for humans, the more complex the machinery, the harder it is to work out why it is not functioning as expected. There are few clean lines, and for many, there is a dizzying fog of possibility around how we came to be.

I think I am lucky with my own experience of life, as I have a story which I think explains a lot about how and why my mind functions as it does. A story, a coherent narrative, is certainly a useful thing to have. It is something to look at, to interrogate. You can poke stories with a stick.

My mother

Before my story, I am going to tell you about the end of someone else's story: my mother's.

My mother was dying, at home, but in a hospital bed. The room

CRASH!

she was dying in was next door to the room I was born in. She was fading out, sometimes quietly and sometimes in great distress. My dad was talking to her in a way that we – my sister and I – had not heard him use before, with different pet names, a different tone. Maybe this was how he had often spoken to her in private, but this was the first time we had heard it. There was an intensity to his voice, a broken-heartedness, a desperate calm in trying to help her escape the nightmare visions. It seemed like he was not talking to the woman she was now, but the woman he first fell in love with.

Fifty years had vanished, and perhaps the young woman she had once been was there again, the one who sought his help and love when she was nineteen years old and still grieving for her lost father. In this moment, I finally understood something enormous that had happened to our family many years before.

It was something that had been in plain sight, yet utterly invisible. It was something that had a huge effect on all of us, but which we decided to treat with silence and busyness.

I heard it in a dream

I was being interviewed in a dream. I often have vivid and bizarre dreams, narratives that run as if directed by Luis Buñuel and starring Peter Cushing and Kenneth Williams holding up a mirror to the ninth dimension, but this was not one of them. This was a plain dream with no special guests.

'When were you born?'

'Seventeenth February 1972.'

This was not my birth date, I first appeared on 20 February 1969, but my dream-world birth date made sense. I think the ME-ness of ME was born on that day in 1972. It was the day of the crash.

Seventy-two hours before my third birthday party, I was in a car accident. I was uninjured, my sister needed three stitches to her scalp, but my mother was seriously hurt and went into a coma. I can still recall the moments after the crash, my confusion and my sister crying and bleeding.

My mother was as still as death.

I was full of sickening guilt.

I was two years, eleven months and twenty-eight days old, and I thought I must have caused the accident. Children often make the link from catastrophe to themselves. It can seem like a form of negative narcissism, but it's actually an attempt to make sense of a difficult, complex and often scary world around them, to protectively give themselves some agency and control. Not only had I caused this accident, I was the cause of all the pain and depression that my mother would go on to battle with.

As I write this, fifty-two years on, the ghosts of that day are still vivid. While some people grow up with the ability to take credit, however little they were involved in a success, others are adept at blaming themselves for pain and failure, however distant from the cause they were.

The more difficulty and trauma in a young child's life, the more the adults around them seem distressed, angry, unhappy, unapproachable, scary, the more a child can retreat into themselves, and blame themselves for the events around them. How much simpler for that child to place the blame for all the chaos and complexity in their life at their own feet than to consider the fact that the world is this terrible, scary and unhappy place. That child must then work harder not to make the world worse; they must hide their own sadness, anxiety, fear and be other than they are – quieter, more pleasing, or more demanding. How many of you reading this now have blamed yourself for your parents' divorce or even the death of a loved one? Minor recriminations can grow into vast haunting forests that overshadow your life.

I first wrote about the car accident in the book *I'm a Joke and So Are You*. I didn't really want to because I was worried that it would be seen as showing off – 'Look at *my* sadness!' – when I knew so

CRASH!

many had experienced far worse. One of my biggest worries then was the possibility of collateral damage to others involved, particularly my dad, who was a widower in his later eighties. I would rather he hadn't read the book, but he did. It was the first time he realized that I had blamed myself for the crash.

He called me shortly before I was to take the stage at a book festival in Bristol. His voice had a catch in it, and I could hear that he was obviously talking around the subject he intended to get to. Then he said, 'I wish I'd known you thought the crash was your fault, then I could have done something about it.'

It broke my heart. He was always a good and kind man, even if he did have a habit of embarrassing us by shouting very loudly at people who parked on the village green or rode horses where they shouldn't. He had been hurled into a terrible situation and had worked hard for all of us.

I explained to him that nothing could have been done. That a three-year-old could not have explained himself. I also told him that he had been the most remarkable parent during the most terrible time. As children, we often lack the knowledge or experience to understand ourselves or our feelings. Now, we might know more about systems to put in place after such incidents, but then, it was 'carry on as best you can, and if you are lucky, a neighbour may bring around a beef stew or an apple crumble while your wife or mother is otherwise engaged with her coma'. The presumption that my dad couldn't cook was very accurate, and I can't really remember what we ate for a while. In retirement, he mastered barbecued bananas with raspberry jam, chocolate and some kind of liqueur. He was very proud of it. Eventually, he could boil eggs without causing explosions too.

After the accident, when she finally came home from hospital, my mother would often become emotionally distressed, and my father could not always reason with her. Sometimes, he would be too exhausted to try. Feeling isolated and abandoned, she would slam the door to her bedroom and weep uncontrollably. Little me would then gently knock on her door, sneak in and try to calm her down and make her happy.

'Mummy, are you alright? Can I do anything?'

She would try to talk through her weeping. Sometimes, my intervention would be enough for her to gather herself up a little and she would talk of her sadness, and we might eventually play Top Trumps Cricketers (either British edition or International). I look back now and realize how lost and scared she was. The further away it is, the more vivid the picture becomes, and my stomach knots whenever I stumble into those memories again.

After I wrote about the crash, a friend encouraged me to go to a therapist for a while. During one session, I came across the ultimate cliché from the 'stand-up comedian documentary' playbook, the heartstring plucking moment where the cellos swell or, due to budgetary restrictions, the electronic keyboard attempts to ape an orchestra.

'So, Robin, why did you become a comedian?'

'I used to try and put on shows to make my depressive mother happy.'

I told you it was a cliché, and I am quite aware that it is a little too neat, but it is a start.

Something else that opened up, since I first wrote about the crash, was understanding how my mother's life-changing injuries affected my older sisters and the family as a whole.

My mother had one lung damaged when her ribs were smashed, her jaw had been shattered, she had had to have a tracheotomy, had lost numerous teeth, had facial paralysis, had lesions in her brain and never regained her sense of smell. That she never lost her ability to cook wonderful treats for us seems remarkable to me.

The really impactful physical damage was to her brain and how that altered her perception of herself. Many years later, when she had to have her brain scanned again, the doctor found it quite incredible that she had survived and had continued to live an active life in any way at all. But she had depression and anxiety for the rest of her life.

The lesions in her brain are what I believe led to her developing dementia in her sixties, though that was not actually diagnosed until it popped up on her death certificate. Social care turned up for the first time to help my dad look after my mum two days after she died. They stayed for a while to dismantle the bed she died in.

Trauma

The understanding of how trauma affects us has greatly increased in the twenty-first century. Almost like the realization that washing your hands before surgery, especially if they are covered in the black blood of your previous patient, may well decrease the chance of passing on infection, the long-term effects of trauma, previously so ignored and unknown, seem now to be so obvious.

I have spoken to a lot of neurodivergent people, and many have had trauma in their background. Childhood disruption can be very important in the development of the brain and in the behaviour patterns we then have as adults. Unfortunately, many, like myself, have spent much of their life dismissing their trauma as not being traumatic enough.

If you know someone who was five when the rest of their family was murdered by a bloodthirsty cult, or someone who was imprisoned down a well until they were fourteen years old, then one car crash and a changed mother seem small beans.*

Perhaps there is an objective scale of terribleness and trauma, but things being worse for others is not a balm for making everything better for you. If you lose a finger in a bizarre gardening accident,

---

* I don't actually know either the well prisoner or the cult victim – or maybe I do, and they've just not come out about it yet.

it doesn't stop the bleeding and pain if your neighbour has accidentally cut off their leg with a scythe. Equally, the perhaps very British response to trauma of being told to 'just forget it and move on', the famous 'stiff upper lip', handily ignores the fact that it is impossible to 'move on' – because you have to move forward with the same brain in your skull that went through the experiences, which in turn have shaped your networks and your behaviour. It was either Confucius or Yogi Bear who said, 'Wherever you go, that's where you are.'

Dr Heather Sequeira is a consultant psychologist specializing in trauma. When she was a child, her father died of a brain tumour. Like toddler me, she presumed that her existence in the world must have been one of the causes of his death. Her conscious brain, that smart, reasoning part of the mind that Heather calls the 'upstairs brain', knew that just couldn't be the case, but beneath that, the 'downstairs brain', through the stress and anxiety it manufactured, would overpower the upstairs brain into believing she was at fault. Day after day, while the brainiest bit of your brain rationally explains why your terrors are not reasonable, the emotional part of your brain takes no notice whatsoever, hampered by its inability to understand a word your upstairs is saying.

Heather believes that this downstairs brain victory drove all sorts of OCD-like behaviours, allowing her to take control of the world around her in any way she could. She had to put things away in ways she felt were lucky for her. She was not able to say certain things to certain people or even speak to certain people. Heather told me that she was a good musician as a child, but stopped playing because one of the thoughts was, *If I ever pass a piano exam, then somebody will die.* 'Of course, back in the seventies and eighties, you couldn't say this to anybody,' she told me. 'I'd probably have been locked up and injected with chlorpromazine.'

I believe many of us carry a quiet madness with us that is not really madness at all, but the common eccentricity of human thinking, some of it benign and some of it malignant. Here is the place where stress builds as you force yourself to remain silent. The fear of being considered mad can drive you mad. And the longer you do that for, the more isolated you can become. She sees this inability to talk to anybody, her need to keep things to herself, as one of the reasons she was sexually abused as a child by a man in a field. She couldn't tell anybody about it and that man almost certainly knew that about her. Guilt makes you believe that you 'get what you deserve'. Concealing yourself makes it easier to feel that you cannot express anguish or tell other people about those who abuse you. These incidents of trauma were crushing for her, and shame inducing. She says that she was fortunate to have a mentality that could remain open to experience. She didn't shut down completely.

While I was speaking to her, Heather grabbed a flip chart and drew a brain dividing it into upstairs and downstairs. The amygdala, the part of the brain that is understood to play a major part in emotional regulation and fear control is below stairs. Trauma, especially in childhood, can affect its regulation. If we see the amygdala as a meter dial ready to give off a warning when fear kicks in and a plan of action may be necessary, the less trauma in childhood, the lower the dial's initial setting – it's starting point may be one. The more trauma felt or experienced in childhood, the more sensitive it is and the further up the dial the initial setting, so the journey to TEN! won't take very long.

For those who have experienced childhood trauma, the alert system can go off in situations that many would travel through without obstacle or interruption. The important element here is that the trauma develops its grip through our silence, both our failure or fear of expressing ourselves and our failure to give space and make ways for others to share and speak up.

I have a friend, abused by his mother as a child, who grew up to be a homeless drug addict and also spent stretches in prison. Yet it was only in his forties that the long-term effects on his mind and the impact of the trauma in his childhood started to be professionally understood, allowing him to begin to think about his life differently.

Another friend suddenly lost her father when she was seven, and her sister was murdered when she was thirty-five. Now, in her fifties, she has an inkling that some of her intense struggle comes from a potentially ADHD mind, which might have developed in her childhood at the time of that first terrible trauma. The father, who was a symbol of safety and permanence to her as a young girl, was suddenly not there any more. How absolutely terrifying. How could she ever feel stable again? How could she ever feel protected and safe again? How could she ever trust a world where such things could happen? So her brain compensated, trying to cope with an overload of emotions, of anger, of sadness, of fear, running at a million miles an hour, considering all the possibilities, working out all the angles, unable to sit quietly with itself, distracting itself. How wonderful, how useful, not to have to sit with the quiet terror of her own existence.

We have to encourage the children who are secretly battling with the past that shaped them to speak up fearlessly and shamelessly. Brushing things under the carpet not only leads to a very bumpy carpet, it also attracts vermin and then they can bite you and that can lead to madness.

Dandelion?

Fear, like so much in our mind, exists on a spectrum.

Free Solo is a documentary about climbers who ascend the sheer cliff faces of mountains without ropes or the slightest safety precautions. It is the kind of documentary about hazardous hobbies that some people can't even begin to watch, never mind actually partake in the sport. It is a high-risk hobby with a high rate of mortality.

So what marks out those risk-takers from me? The answer is in the brain and particularly the amygdala. The amygdala is where our brains monitor and alert us to what we should be fearful of. Many

CRASH!

free climbers have amygdalae that don't fire when other people's would. The part of the brain that fortunately stops most of us from engaging in excessive jeopardy does not act as a warning system to the free climber. Their fearlessness is more unconsciously biological than consciously psychological.

I went abseiling *once*. I will never have to update that sentence. It is one of the many experiences that have made me aware that my amygdala is in rude health.

It is all very well to say 'fear is something that you have to overcome', but some people have a lot more to overcome than others. Paediatrician W. Thomas Boyce has studied such differences and puts children into two groups, as either being 'dandelions' or 'orchids'. His studies show 80 per cent of children are dandelions, resilient to most environments, while 20 per cent are orchids, who have higher potential but greater fragility. As Boyce puts it, 'The orchid child is the child who shows great sensitivity and susceptibility to both bad and good environments in which he or she finds herself or himself.'[1] I was introduced to these ideas while talking to the author and therapist Philippa Perry who, as I spoke about my childhood, piped up, 'Ah, you are an orchid.'

One of the issues of being an orchid is that your sensitivity gives power to others. The bullies are good at spotting the sensitive and crush them in order to increase their sense of power. But, as we see with bullying figures like Donald Trump, their relentlessness and shamelessness comes from having intense sensitivity for themselves and no one else. The very existence of anyone who may not revere them makes them feel like Joan of Arc. But something that is common among a certain type of bully is the inability or the wish to imagine the pain of others. There are those who want to break anything that distracts from them. They must hate the beautiful for it might interfere with the reflection in their narcissistic pool. They must despise and belittle anything whose needs may distract from theirs.

Our empathy, our concern for ourselves, our worry for others, is also on a spectrum. The kindness of some and the cruelty of others can seem inexplicable. My stomach contracts when I hear a child crying at the unfairness of it all or the pain they are in, whether it's been caused by a knee colliding with the pavement or a lost balloon. I can be overwhelmed, even though I know that often it will be over soon and a new mood will assail them, because in that moment, I can feel the intensity of their despair. Somewhere in trauma-wiring is a connection to another's trauma when you hear or see it.

It is not the right of others to declare whether your trauma is enough to be traumatic or not, just as we cannot state definitively how much pain someone is in after they have trodden on a tack. For many years I was dismissive of the effect of the car crash and everything that followed for me. When I finally faced it full on and the impact that I believe accompanied it, my life and the understanding of it hugely improved. It didn't make me 'needy' as some like to frame any honesty about pain, but it did begin to give me the tools to help me to understand myself.

Executive function

Neurodivergent minds can struggle with both the inevitability of disorder and the desperate need for increased and intense order. For some minds, mine being one, the speed of thoughts is so fast that it can be impossible to complete a task, as every time you go to do that task, the journey to that task generates new ideas and new tasks. All emails over one-sentence long are mainly wasted words. Too many instructions short-circuit me. If I'm being asked to do something then I often need all permutations ironed out into a single route, with all the possibilities carefully ordered.

We are still in the early days of understanding what does what in the human brain, but we have come to some broad understanding of the compartments where various things take place. Sometimes

CRASH!

dubbed 'the personality centre', the prefrontal cortex, the front part of the frontal lobe, is where we process emotions and order information – two of the things that ADHD people battle with.[2] It is posited that trauma affects the prefrontal cortex, and it is believed that childhood stress can disrupt neural circuits and impair development.

Our executive functions are housed in the prefrontal cortex. The 'executive function' of our brains includes the ability to think flexibly, our self-control and our working memory. Our working memory is what allows us to keep track of tasks we are doing as we take in information. As anyone who is ADHD or knows someone who is can tell you, organization and order are not strong points. Focusing and the ease with which the mind can drift from the task at hand are problematic. 'Drift' doesn't even feel like an emphatic enough word. 'Mind-lurching' may be better, and it may be the reason you have reread this page three times.

You might have started concentrating on the words, but then been distracted by the words 'executive function' making your mind wander to the Steven Seagal film, *Executive Decision*, which made you think about The Motors number four hit single 'Airport' and now you're in the kitchen looking for Jaffa cakes and wondering where exactly you have left that book you were just reading. I can wait. I like Jaffa cakes too.

The neural networks of the prefrontal cortex are what brings control to the confusion of existence, and the less well those networks function the greater your anxiety. In *Executive Function and Dysfunction*, authors Scott J. Hunter and Elizabeth Sparrow define the executive functions as a set of:

> '... *interdependent, progressively acquired, higher-order cognitive skills that emerge ... across early childhood, through adolescence, and into early adulthood. Because the development of neural systems that support executive function is so protracted, it*

NORMALLY WEIRD AND WEIRDLY NORMAL

is vulnerable across time to alterations in its unfolding trajectory, resulting in multiple possible routes to executive dysfunction'.[3]

Other papers have stressed how important the prefrontal cortex is in regulating behaviour and how 'deficits' in this area can be disastrous for our psychological wellbeing.[4]

This happened to me as I was writing this chapter.

It was a Wednesday afternoon and, while typing, I broke off to check some details for an event the following day in Chelmsford, about 60 miles from where I live. I would be talking with the author Sarah Perry. It was a 6.30 p.m. start, but not tomorrow, TODAY! I do not drive a car. The train would take at least two hours. My brain goes insane. There is an electrical storm inside my head so strong it could have revived the flesh that Victor Frankenstein stitched.

First, there is panic mode. I phone a nearby friend with a car, but he is not answering.*

My brain won't give me the cab number that I know off by heart.

014444265

01224862

0144286 . . .

Eventually, I recall the number.

I am relentlessly screeching, 'Jesus Christ! Oh my God! F*** F*** F***! Aaaargh! YOU IDIOT!' The rest of my family hide.

The taxi will be ten minutes.

Time slows as if I am falling into a black hole.

I AM.

I had not prepared the interview or finished reading Sarah's novel. I simmered and bubbled in the taxi, then ran the final few hundred metres into the bookshop with one minute to spare. I said hello to Sarah and apologized profusely, and then, in front of sixty people,

---

* It turned out I rang the wrong Charlie – I rang the one who had died, and whose number was still in my phone.

CRASH!

we had a fluent conversation covering faith, ghosts, astronomy and critical failure. The speed from being a brain of despair and confusion to being a brain of full engagement with access to all the knowledge I needed was almost dizzying. The very faults that led to me getting the day wrong, and then being appalling around the house, were also what allowed me to then access exactly what I needed to grasp this defeat and turn it into victory (even if I was quite out of pocket from the taxi fare).

Would that meltdown have happened if that little boy, fifty-two years ago, had not been in a crash that he thought was his fault? I don't think so. But he also wouldn't have grown into the person who could sit in a bookshop discussing the nature of deities and supernovae either.

It seems that childhood trauma can also come from the experience of being ASD, rather than being the cause itself. Or perhaps I should say: the trauma often comes from being ASD and the outside world's reaction to that. According to research from Dr Freya Rumball at King's College London, the rates of probable PTSD in autistic people is between 32 per cent and 45 per cent while it is 4–4.5 per cent in the general population.[5] The research indicates that autistic people may be more likely to experience traumatic life events, particularly interpersonal traumas such as bullying and physical and sexual abuse.

According to Connor Kerns, assistant professor of psychology at the University of British Columbia, about 70 per cent of kids with autism will have a co-morbid psychiatric disorder.

I only learned the rather gloomy term 'comorbidity' as I went on my neurodivergent adventure. However, it is not as gloomy as it sounds – it simply refers to the presence of two or more conditions within one person. As we'll find out later on, there are many neurodivergent people who possess more than one neurodivergence within the current parameters. And if we don't find out more later on, that is because I totally forgot my promise of telling you more due to my ADHD. My editor will probably remind me, though, as he reckons he is not neurodivergent, so is without a cast-iron alibi.

Expectations

Traumatic childhood experiences can also transform one's expectations of the world. The more upsets and disturbances that deviate from a contented life that one experiences as a child, the more suspicions might grow about reality and its possibilities. Each time you experience a threat from the world, it increases your wariness. Your sense of impending doom becomes fine-tuned.

The more I thought about the crash and its impact over the following years of my childhood and beyond, the more certain patterns of behaviour I had engaged in made sense.

I have had a terrible fear of making people unhappy – again, perhaps connected to that unhappiness that I believe I caused my mother. In any room with other people, I would worry that I was making them unhappy or just not being good enough. The limited access I had to that prefrontal cortex meant that emotions, particularly negative emotions, had too much control.

Are you alright? Are you angry? Is it my fault? Have I ruined the day? These were the thoughts of a small boy who believed he had done something terrible and caused such unhappiness he never wanted to be the cause of such sadness again. Frequently, ADHD people I meet describe how, before diagnosis, they really wanted to make people happy, even if the effort involved brought pain to themselves. And when they did make people happy, they soon found a way to not believe that they had genuinely achieved anything, or they found that the moment could bring with it a sense of failure or shame. After diagnosis, this desire to please and connect does not go away, but at least the inevitability of failure starts to fade.

CRASH!

Talking

Since I started writing about my past and the crash, my sisters and I have started talking about what happened to us all. We rarely talked about such things when we were growing up. I don't really remember any discussion in my childhood beyond being told to wait in the car when my mum and dad went into psychiatric evaluations and then the excitement of receiving £40 damages all to myself after the five-year trial led by Lord Denning (it was exceptionally long as we were one of five cases that were being reviewed in the hope of changing judicial process). I wanted to splash out on an Action Man assault course, but I think the money was put in my Post Office account . . .

I must find out what I did with the savings books. I might have accrued a fortune, perhaps enough to buy a new rake. Certainly not enough to buy an Action Man assault course, as they are very collectable now and way out of my price range. In fact, looking back, the best investment would have been splashing out on the Action Man assault course and never opening it. Oh, the Monaco hotels I could be reclining in . . .

It wasn't forbidden to talk about the crash, we just didn't. So I am glad we are beginning to do so now. I have no memories of my mother before the crash. Like the dream I had, my life, or the memory of it, begins, or seems to, just after the collision. My sisters said that they thought it was sad that I have no memories of who Mum was before, but in other ways, I think I am fortunate. I have no comparison. I don't know what I lost, only what I had.

They have also told me a little more about the things I did not see.

I sit with my eldest sister, Janey, in the kitchen of the house we grew up in. This is where our mum baked those chocolate cakes and flapjacks. When sadder memories of her life start to dominate, I force myself to recall licking the last gooey remnants of raw cake mix from the mixing bowl. I can picture the orange sponge mix on the end the wooden spoon and I can taste it too. My Proust sponge cake moment.

This is also the kitchen where our mum, during one of her lowest ebbs and at the height of her mental turmoil, went to stab our father with a screwdriver. Eventually, the screwdriver went through a pane of glass in the window instead. The hole in the window lasted for most of our childhood, a piece of plastic sellotaped over it. It was a convenient hole for us to sneak our small hands through so we could break into the house when no one was home.

My eldest sister was nine years old at the time of the crash. She was at home watching *Top of the Pops*, which that week had mimed performances by Slade, The Sweet and Chicory Tip, as well as Cliff Richard singing a song called 'Jesus' in which he implores Jesus to come back to Earth. It has a nice brass arrangement but only gained a low chart position, so in future years, Cliff kept to just talking about Jesus and lowered his biblical disco output.

My dad rang home, perhaps between Harry Nilsson's 'Without You' and Billy Preston's 'I Wrote a Simple Song', and told my sister that there had been a bit of an accident, but it was fine, just cuts and bruises. This was a white lie. None of us children had any knowledge of the extent of our mother's injuries at the time. I imagine my sisters were expecting Mum would be home by the end of the week.

A couple of days later, my sister drew a card with a horse on it and wrote on the other side:

Dear Mummy,
* I want to see you soon. We had Robin's party on Saturday, it was a great success. Hope to see you as soon as I can.*
* LOTS OF LOVE LOVE LOVE LOVE LOVE*
* From Janie.*
* PS I did NOT trace the horse.*

CRASH!

To remove all doubt, her friend Rosanda wrote 'TRUE' or rather 'TURE'.

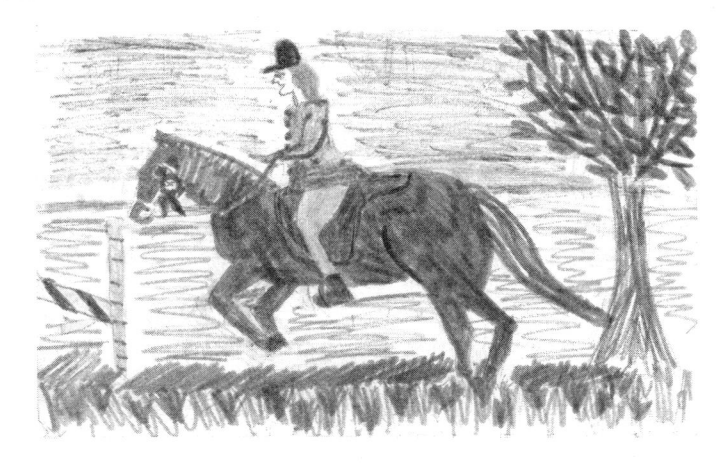

When my dad returned from the hospital, he told Janey that Mum had loved the card. Really, she hadn't seen it. She was still in a coma.

Many weeks later, none of us remember quite how many, Mum left hospital. Sarah and Janey hid in the bushes and watched her return. They were worried.

Who would they meet?

What would they see?

I don't think any of us had imagined how changed she would be. Dad led her very slowly down the garden path, her jaw in a metal frame, her memory of where she was and who we all were less than certain. It is an event I don't believe I witnessed, but my non-memory has recreated the scene. I can see what I never saw.

We were all taken up individually to see her in her bed. What must we have thought? Janey told me that Mum didn't recognize her, but she did recognize Sarah and me.

Her recovery was long and hard. Our GP, Dr Webber, was a man considered a saint by my family. Not only was he a good GP, but when I was being born one snowy evening, he brought with him a snow shovel so he could dig his way into the snowbound village and get to the birth. Yet even he told my father that he thought it had reached the point where my mum should be sectioned. The advice was that she should be put in a residential home and my father should 'move on with his life'.

My father was having none of that. His vow, both of marriage and of love, meant that he would support her whatever happened. For all the confusion of looking back at my childhood, one thing that has grown stronger and stronger with age is the realization of just how admirable he was.

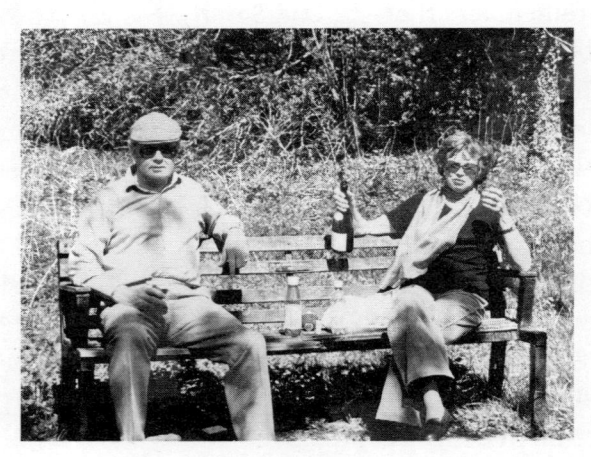

My parents looking like rural gangsters.

Years later, when someone told my dad what an amazing man he was because so many men would have just left their wife, he was perplexed at the idea that he could or would have done anything differently. In a book about being 'weird', it is perhaps worth making clear how odd I find it that my dad's commitment to my mother has been considered by many to have not been the normal way.

As grotesque as it may sound, a doctor told me that the general way of things when a woman experienced a life-changing injury was that, after a few months, the husband would move on. I am glad that

CRASH!

my dad was weirder than other men of that time, that his 'weirdness' was a weirdness of love and devotion.

Mum started to recover and her behaviour became more stable, but she battled with depression and coming to terms with how her circumstances had changed and who she was. The first time my dad had to go away after the accident, on a twenty-four-hour business trip, she locked herself in a bedroom and said she would jump out of the window if he left. He drove away anyway. He knew he had to call this particular bluff, but I know he would have been agonizing about it. She remained in the bedroom.

Janey remembers that she and Sarah would sit at the top of the stairs listening to our parents having blazing rows, wondering if they might need to step in and 'save Dad'. On one occasion, a blazing row did lead to actual flames when cushions were thrown into the fire, followed by more agonized weeping and slammed doors. On another occasion, when my father had to go abroad, Mum started faking a heart attack. She was filled with anxiety and, I think, genuinely terrified that, because she was not quite as she had been in the past, Dad would leave her.

Talking to my eldest sister recently, I told her I would lie in bed listening to the rows, hoping Mum and Dad would get divorced. I would dream of being adopted by the actor Christopher Lee whose horror films I loved so much and going to live with him in LA, though perhaps living at the seaside with Peter Cushing would have been the better option.

As a child, I would often have my own meltdowns. At my own birthday parties, I would burst into tears and run away and hide in the cupboard under the stairs if I lost one of the party games. But I'd never do this at someone else's birthday party. I could just about accept failing to be the one to unwrap a bar of Fruit and Nut at other people's parties. Maybe it was because I didn't know if they had a cupboard under the stairs I could run off to.

I also remember bursting into tears over my ugliness and

becoming so full of rage that I would smash doors and cupboards. To an adult, such behaviour can seem like wilful brattishness, deserving of punishment, being shouted at or sent to your bedroom. Parents may have limited resources to deal with what can be considered 'bad behaviour', but not all brats are really brattish. Sadly, some proverbs of the Bible have stuck more than others, and we still live in a world that feels that sparing the rod will spoil the child, perhaps because beating is far simpler than talking and understanding. To be fair to the Bible, in this instance it only states, 'He that spareth his rod hateth his son: but he that loveth him chasteneth him betimes,' and it was the seventeenth-century poet Samuel Butler who added the spoiling of the child.

Sports were also quite impossible for me, as every time I fumbled, fell or dropped, my head would explode with rage at myself for being so damn lousy. I came to realize that I was safest, and happiest, when I was alone with just my comic books for company.

For both ASD and ADHD people, emotional regulation is difficult. The speed from peace to meltdown can be frighteningly fast. Dr Heather Sequeira describes this as 'somatic sensory processing dysfunction', the way the body responds to trauma, sometimes years down the line. She explains that 'this can lead to challenges in physiological arousal modulation and regulation of emotion'. Sensory sensitivity plays a major part in many neurodivergent minds, and this is also increasingly being linked to traumatic experience. Experience of childhood trauma appears to create higher levels of sensory sensitivity, which has been researched using self-report measures of centralized pain. It has also been shown that traumatic brain injury (TBI) can change sensory processing, which would go part of the way to explaining my mother's extreme reactions and sensitivity in many situations.

People experiencing PTSD can experience changes in visual processing at a pre-attentive level. The pre-attentive level is the subconscious level, where much of the environmental input is taken in and processed and only what is considered important makes it into your conscious awareness. For those whose subconscious has been modified by trauma, there can be a heightened anxiety to what others would find mundane or perhaps not even have been made aware of in the first place.

Somatic sensory processing dysfunction, when it is at the brain-stem level, can impact the arousal of fear, anxiety and fight or flight responses. This heightened sense of stress and tension can lead to anger, lashing out and a loss of control.

The more I have spoken to friends openly about their battles with mental health, the more I have found out how many have had traumatic experiences in childhood. In a more enlightened world, they would have been able to talk about these experiences, helped to understand how they were suffering from PTSD and felt heard and cared for, all of which might have alleviated some of the anxiety and pain around such feelings. But most were left to 'just get on with it', expected to leave it behind them. Yet, to stress again, you cannot just leave the events of your life behind you as if you were just moving house.

I have friends who have lost parents in violent circumstances, had guns held to their head when they were seven years old and experienced psychological and physical abuse from adults, and all of them have just kept moving forward, seeing the difficulties they had getting through life as their own fault and something to try to bury as deeply as possible. In their paper 'The brain–body disconnect: A somatic sensory basis for trauma-related disorders', brain scientists Kearney and Lanius explain how 'an altered neural defense circuitry leading to persistent sensory and emotional overwhelm in response to stimuli is evident in trauma-related disorders'.[6]

A common rejoinder is that 'it's no good dwelling in the past', but successfully dwelling in the present can often be greatly helped by understanding your past and those who made it.

NORMALLY WEIRD AND WEIRDLY NORMAL

Shame

I see my short temper and highly strung nature as very possibly being connected to shame.

Sometimes, my mum and I would set each other off. Getting back one day from a day out in London with my mum, she couldn't find the door key. Her frustration made me frustrated. I probably needed the toilet or I was just being an impatient child. She became angry, and as we wound each other up, she cut her face on a rose branch that was hanging over the door. She exploded. I hadn't meant to be bad and ruin the day. I started saying sorry over and over again, but she dragged me into the outside toilet and locked me in. At least I now had somewhere cold and rusty to wee. I remember banging on the door and pleading with her, and feeling so bad. That is another memory that knots my stomach each time I return to it.

The catalogue of memories that I feel ashamed of is as thick and tatty as anything you might find in a monastery library. One such silly non-infraction came after my dad took me to *Star Wars*. He bought me a treat at my request, a poster magazine, but then, in the car, I realized I had pointed out the wrong one. This was poster magazine number two, the one with Han, Chewie, Obi Wan and Luke in the Millennium Falcon cockpit, and I had meant to get number one. I started to obsess about it being wrong. Eventually, that eight-year-old wound up his dad so much that he stopped at the traffic lights turned around to me in the back seat and tore the magazine to shreds. Unlike my sister's Donnie Osmond poster, this one was never sellotaped back together again.

The guilt returns to me every time I think of it. My dad, under tremendous pressure in his life, takes his son out and then his son won't stop whining about a bloody poster of a Jedi and a Wookiee (maybe C-3PO was there too). I went to stay with my grandmother that night. I remember I was seething about how much I hated my dad, though really, I hated myself for not just being a boy who said

CRASH!

thank you. It's a silly little story, a tiny moment in a whole childhood, and yet its emotional weight still hangs heavily and I can tangibly feel the pain and guilt around it in middle age. Emotional recall doesn't necessarily shrink as the years after incidents increase.

Perhaps after the trauma of the crash and its impact, it was easy to turn quibbles into traumatic events. My dial was turned up way too high, sensitive and alert to any threat, but I had no control over the setting or even where I kept my thermostat. For all of this, my thoughts of running away, my hatred of the arguments my parents would have, my desperate wish for peace, the blame I projected onto myself, I did not actually want to be detached from my family. I was filled with love for them and saw myself as the problem.

Show me a picture of my mother, I can instantly tell if it was before or after the crash, even if it is in profile and shows the side of her face that did not suffer the tell-tale nerve damage. There was a happy-go-luckiness she had before that was stolen by what happened.

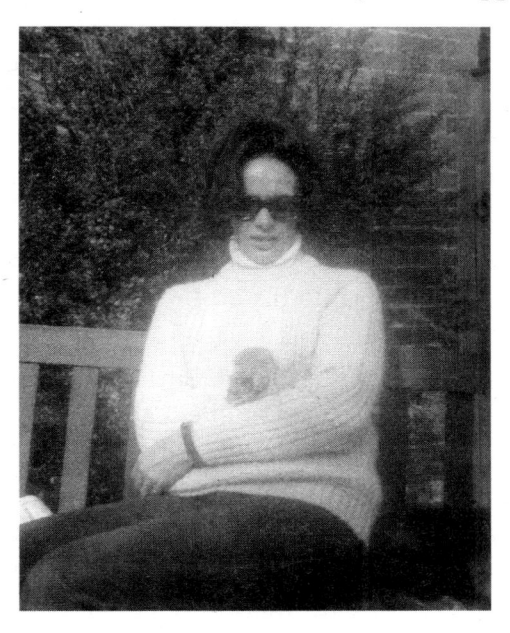

Probably the last photograph of our mum before the accident.

NORMALLY WEIRD AND WEIRDLY NORMAL

At the Wigtown Book Festival, I saw the activist and writer Natasha Walter talking about a book she had written about her mother. Her mother had taken her own life at seventy-five years old, worried that she was developing dementia. Natasha knew why she did it and respected that she was someone who had wanted to be in control of her destiny. When her interviewer asked if she thought her mother would have been happy to have been written about, she replied that she believed her mother had deliberately left clues and notes so that her life could be pieced together. Halfway through the book, her mother is no longer called Mother and Natasha calls her Ruth, because Natasha now knows the human being who was Ruth, the human being she didn't see when Ruth was just 'Mother'.

The longer it has been since my mother died, the more I wish I had asked her questions about how she felt about things, about her state of mind. She experienced depression for most of my life. As far as I know, this was all because of the car accident. The more I look at photographs from before the crash, the more I wonder about the mother I never knew. The more I look at photographs from after the crash, the more I wish I had talked more with the mother that I did know. Sadly, I don't believe my sisters or I will ever know Pamela, but I believe that wishing we could have known her is a good start.

Perhaps as the generations change, the gap that was there in the past is not as clearly defined as it once was. For many, there is no longer the border wall that was traditionally built between parent and child – the hierarchies that meant it would be impolite to talk equally, to enquire of an elder how they really were. The taboos preventing us from asking them about what has so often been kept secret are perhaps being dismantled.

One such taboo is neurodivergence. Many people grow up in neurodivergent families and never know it, often because no one else in the family realizes that they are neurodivergent. We paper over the cracks in our minds and just keep going, smiling broadly while secretly despairing.

CRASH!

Top of the Pops

The hardest part about writing this chapter was when I discovered the listing for *Top of the Pops* for 17 February 1972. It wasn't hard to find, but I'd never searched before and finding it made the day of the crash seem very real, not just something in the jumble of my memory. The evening my mother was terribly injured in a car crash, changing all of our lives for ever, was an evening when my nine-year-old sister was waiting to see Slade on our boxy old black-and-white television.

I am someone who has an unhealthy need to control his emotions, someone who would not allow himself to cry at either of his parents' funerals, even though that is the place where tears are permitted and even considered excusable by the English. I made it through both eulogies intact enough to worry if this was just another sign that I was actually a psychopath.

But then something suddenly jumps out at you.

As I read the listing for that *Top of the Pops*, I could feel the weight that builds up around the eye, the one that says 'you are dangerously close to an emotional experience'. I told my family about the listing, but the catch in my throat soon made me return to my attic study. I wrote myself away from the scene.

I believe I am good at talking about other people's emotions. I am not embarrassed by other people crying, and I will do as much as possible to be available and helpful to people experiencing distress, but this does not work for myself. Psychiatrist Dr Anya Borissova sees it as a common but strange contradiction that makes sense from an ancient human perspective. Sharing your own emotions is exposing. You need to be comfortable with being vulnerable. Much like being secretive with a therapist, handing over what is frequently societally defined as weakness can feel threatening. Though it is possible we evolved to cry and look sad in order to signal that we needed help, unfortunately, shame gets in the way. I think the inability to openly display sadness is about shame, and that is not something that is easy to shift.

But it can also be alienating for people if you are unable to ask for help. My wife has only ever seen me cry a couple of times, once while I was watching *The Elephant Man* (because I hadn't noticed her entering the room) and once during a particularly moving episode of *Inside No. 9*. Being 'strong' can be a trap. Your partner gets used to your inability to ask for help or to cry, and then suddenly, after almost a decade of boxing it all up, you burst into tears, and they just think that you have gone quite mad.

I also found that my brain became paralysed when I was writing about the argument I had with my mother which led to her being cut by the rose bush. I got such a vivid sense of her and her battles and how hard those battles could be and how much she felt she had lost when she woke up from her coma. That is why I think it is important to tell you what an incredible spirit she was, how hard she fought, and how good her George Washington American Ginger Cake was. She was wonderful with the dogs she looked after when we didn't need looking after any more, and she loved our father and he loved her.

Watching my favourite TV show, *Mr Inbetween*, there is a scene between Ray, the smart and impenetrable hitman, and his dad, now suffering from dementia and in a care home. Their relationship has been broken for many years, but Ray's father must tell him something. He talks of being a soldier in Vietnam, of returning home to be told that he was a baby-killer, and how the strain and guilt destroyed him. He looks at Ray and says, 'I wish you'd known me before I went to war.' How that sentence hits.

Trauma can twist and break and change you, until you aren't really you any more. I would have liked to have known my mother before she went to her war. Perhaps there is someone you wish knew you before they went to their war or you went to yours.

2. WEIRDO OR WHEN DID YOU REALIZE YOU WERE ODD?

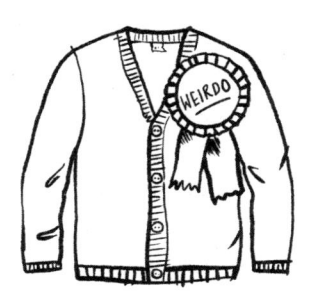

I wear a badge which reads, 'Weirdo'. I probably don't need to wear it, as my face most likely projects that message of its own accord. But some days I attach the badge to my cardigan so there can be no doubt, to make sure no one jumps to any false assumptions about me. While I am aware that my middle-aged white male in a cardigan look severely reduces the chances of being hassled about my appearance, anyone approaching me has no one to blame but themselves, should they become burdened by an idiosyncratic conversation.

I wear the badge in memory of Sophie Lancaster and in the hope of creating a world that is safer for the weird, for those who stand out enough for other people to want to strike them down. In some places, it doesn't take much for people to want to punish you for your existence. Sometimes it just takes the form of persistent verbal abuse, or creating an atmosphere of threat, but sometimes it is murder.

Sophie was beaten to death when she was twenty years old. The perpetrators were reported to have shouted 'WEIRDO!' 'MOSHER!' 'FREAK!' as they attacked her and her boyfriend.* Her mother,

---

* I have not named her boyfriend, as I believe he is attempting to continue with his life as best he can.

NORMALLY WEIRD AND WEIRDLY NORMAL

Sylvia, set up the Sophie Lancaster Foundation, which is an anti-bullying organization that visits institutions including prisons and schools. She uses the brutal murder of her daughter to try to make people understand that to appear different is not to be wrong. Indeed, some of those who strike out do so because they are desperately hiding their own weirdness and see lashing out as a way of proclaiming themselves 'normal'. By punching 'the odd child', they are declaring, 'I am not like that . . . honest. How could I be? I just kicked it.'

Many people have the idea that they are weird thrust upon them. We might live in blissful ignorance of our difference for the first few years of our lives, but then it is in the institutions of our society, such as schools or prisons or at work, where we often discover that we are 'not as others'.

It doesn't take much to be weird. Weirdness often comes at a stage in life when the social rules begin to solidify and self-awareness gives you a mirror that means, when you look at yourself, you start to see your reflection as being like a circus sideshow poster. It has nothing to do with weakness, and it is frequently about the accidental disobedience of failing to conform to a set of rules that you had no part in creating; you may well not understand why they exist at all.

If you have been fortunate or privileged enough to not have had the pressure of social rules and expectations thrust too severely upon you in the first few years of life, school is where these rules and expectations become unavoidably evident. Learning to avoid doing anything that is going to make you stand out unnecessarily is more important than learning your times tables or how to spell 'necessarily'. The slightest slip might generate an unkind and irreversible nickname and reputation.

Reputations are easy to gain and hard to shift. There could be just one incident when you call the teacher 'Mummy' or your swimming trunks slide off as you get out of the pool and then you are burdened

WEIRDO or WHEN DID YOU REALIZE YOU WERE ODD?

until graduation with taunts of 'MUMMY'S BOY!' or 'BUMMY!', or 'MUMMY BUM BUM!' if you are unlucky enough for both incidents to have taken place. Sadly, some never grow out of the belief that a nickname can tarnish someone, and it can be seen being put to pathetic use in modern politics.

You don't even need to say or do anything unusual. It could be your religion, ethnicity or accent that marks you out. Or the radar of the status quo might pick up on the loose threads of your jumper or a vaguely shambolic walking style, and so you are identified as not being part of the alpha pack. A true alpha pack would have no need for bullying or nicknames, as they would have the confidence to be themselves without standing on others to gain height. This is *The Lord of the Flies* model of existence: making someone the runt so others can feel more powerful.

Silly fat cow

Octavia is a qualified therapist who, during her training, discovered she was ADHD and then, a little later, that she was also on the autistic spectrum. There was an ADHD boy at school when she was growing up and he climbed all over the desks and made merry hell during the lessons, whereas she was just told off for playing with her hair and fidgeting a lot. Octavia didn't call her teacher 'Mummy', but she did call her something that created a reaction and a long-term impact.

She vividly recalls being slapped by her teacher when she was ten years old. Her teacher had lost some of Octavia's work and had told her to do it again. Octavia, quite rightly, felt this was very unreasonable. It was not *her* fault. Having a strong antenna for injustice is something many neurodivergent people carry with them. It is hard to just roll over and accept 'the rules' if they don't seem to make sense or don't seem fair. Neurodivergent people can experience unjust admonishment more often and more acutely than their peers, because of the difficulty they have in just sitting silently when they perceive injustice to themselves or others.

On this occasion, Octavia sat back down and said under her breath, 'Silly fat cow.' The boy sitting next to her looked shocked and said, 'I'm going to tell,' and Octavia replied, 'Go on then.'

'Miss! Octavia just called you a "silly fat cow".'

She was told to come to the front and the teacher asked her, 'What did you say?' And Octavia thought, *Well, I have to tell the truth*. 'I called you a silly fat cow.' And that's when the teacher hit Octavia. And then she said, 'I'm going to call your mother.' Her mother didn't have a house phone, so Octavia said, 'Well, that's going to be difficult because we don't have a phone.' And the teacher hit her again.

One problematic task for many neurodivergent people is learning to be dishonest. Much of society prefers the simplicity of dishonesty as opposed to the complexity of the truth. For years, Octavia never quite understood what happened that day in that classroom when her teacher hit her. She now knows what she said had sounded like sass, but for her, at the time, she was just voicing the facts. It was only when she got her diagnosis that she understood who this wise-cracking ten-year-old really was.

A classroom is a room constructed around strict rules and hierarchies, and as a result, anything deviating from the 'norm' can be considered as weird.

'Why can't you sit still?!'

Sitting still sounds like the easiest thing in the world for people who sit still. Stillness is the natural state of rest for many people, but not for many people with ASD or ADHD. To an ADHD mind, sitting still is impossible and boring. It builds up tension. Where is the reward and what is the point? Where does it say that being still is the best way to learn?

WEIRDO or WHEN DID YOU REALIZE YOU WERE ODD?

As an adult, I was once told off for being too active on the quiet coach of a train to Edinburgh. I wasn't using my phone or listening to music, I was just moving too much, picking up too many different books and putting them down again and typing too enthusiastically. I often have one leg that can appear to be pumping a portable organ during Methodist musical worship, and perhaps I was doing that on that carriage that day.

My fidgeting at school was perpetual doodling as well as chewing the paper of my exercise books, so I always ended up with fewer pages than everyone else to fill. I lived in fear of being told off, so all my disobedience was carefully hidden. I was also one of those kids who was always bursting to answer the teacher's questions, the one who almost ripped their arm out of their socket as they thrust their hand in the air with a 'ME! ME! ME!' I was perpetually seeking validation, constantly wanting something to happen. But a good child is a still child, and a bad child is a fidgety child. 'Why can't you be more like Nancy? Look at how still and upright she sits while you slouch and wriggle.'

For many ASD people, what others see as fidgeting can actually be defined as 'stimming' (self-stimulating behaviour). Such behaviour may help calm someone down, or distract them, or relieve stress. This could be jiggling feet, or scratching, or regularly clearing their throat or biting nails.* Stimming can also include flapping your arms when excited by an idea, or needing to mutter constantly. None of these things should disturb other people, but in a world where there are so many regulations about what is supposedly acceptable and normal, some of these actions can disturb people because any sense of otherness is deemed a threat, and again, this is particularly heightened in that crucible of conformity, the classroom. I have observed this as a performer. Sometimes, I hear noise

---

* As horrible as it may sound to you, I have never had to use nail clippers – sorry! My fingernails are usually dentally trimmed to the quick.

from within an audience and I will usually be able to work out to some degree of accuracy whether it is just the sound of neurodivergent stimming or someone clearing their throat, so I know not to be distracted or confrontational.

'Look me in the eyes when I am speaking to you!'

Another failure of conformity is not looking into a teacher's eyes as they talk to you. This can specifically penalize ASD kids. Meeting someone's gaze is considered a physical sign of paying attention, of being empathic, of listening to the other person attentively. In short, it is considered a sign of being socially well-behaved. I dispute this.

From my perspective, I am very good at looking directly into people's eyes, though much of that time is spent not listening to a word they say because my internal monologue is checking on whether I am looking in their eyes too much, whether I should reduce the time I am looking in their eyes, whether I should comment on the sleep dust that is clinging to their eyelashes, whether my face appears wise enough or too earnest as they are speaking, whether I misinterpreted a sad story as a joke and smiled at the wrong time, while also worrying if I've got a sesame seed caught in my teeth which might fly out and land on their iced bun when I open my mouth to pretend I have understood what they just said.

Lack of eye contact is a well-established common signifier for autism, so much so that Annelies, whose son, River, is autistic, was told by a stranger that River is not autistic because he looked people in the eye. River explained that he had learned it as a trick to aid his social conformity. He would concentrate on the bridge of people's noses as that created the illusion of looking them in the eye. This is a good example of someone learning a skill not to improve their life but to mask their own discomfort to make others feel comfortable.

WEIRDO or WHEN DID YOU REALIZE YOU WERE ODD?

'Pay attention when I am speaking!'

Paying attention is defined as doing nothing but staring at whoever is taking the lesson or delivering the annual shareholders' presentation on pork belly investments. For some, creating the appearance of paying attention ultimately creates exactly the opposite situation inside their head. When River went to university and started attending lectures, he would listen, but he would read a novel simultaneously, as this actually helped the information sink in. If he just tried to listen, he found the delivery too slow and he couldn't focus. As Annelies described it, 'He had to use half his brain to do something entirely different so he could type in the information.'

I have to explain to people that I am listening to what they are saying, even though I am doing something else. I am actually able to listen to them more intensely when I am doing something else. I am not distracted by Squaredle and the fury of not being able to find the last twelve-letter word, I am in fact caught in a word conundrum so that the words you are saying to me are less jumbled to my mind. 'Ah! It was "haberdashers"! . . . But on the subject of your opinion on the behaviour of the blobfish . . .' This is an example of one of the many processes where there is more than one way of doing it, which many people really cannot comprehend and get very cross about.

As odd as it may seem, the appearance of total concentration may be quite the opposite. Perpetual doodling, for instance, is not necessarily a sign of switching off, but a sign of someone fighting to maintain attention. An overactive racing mind does not always take well to focusing on just one thing. It seeks and needs constant stimulation and surprise.

The opening scene of Todd Solondz's *Welcome to the Dollhouse* may well cause anxious flashbacks for a filmgoer. Dawn Wiener is a geeky girl in heavy-framed glasses, at a time before spectacles became so fashionable that kids now pray for myopia. These were the days of 'specky four-eyes', where spectacles were yet another way of demoting you to the gamma crowd. She is walking through the school canteen looking for a safe space to sit. Each table holds threats or rejection. You can feel the knot in her stomach. I watched it with my friend Justine. We were surrounded by people laughing at the situation, but Justine and I weren't laughing. We were recalling our own canteen hell.

'Canteen hell' is still a short-cut trope for high school movies to convey the isolation of being odd. Is there nowhere to sit and eat your cheeseburger and fries (or hairy mashed potato and semolina in the UK version)? Nowhere else will you discover just how far out from the in-crowd you are than in the school dining room. It's a trope that continues into adulthood with that other Hollywood staple, the prison drama. Are you the loser who sits with other losers, or are you so lost, so much of an outsider, that you sit in total isolation?

I think school became truly stressful for me when I was around eight and a half, when I moved from the village school to a fee-paying school. It was there that my outcast days truly began. Firstly, I was a newcomer. BAD. Secondly, I was not very well co-ordinated. Not being good at sport is BAD. The ability to throw and catch is revered at school as much as if we still needed such skills in order to chase and kill woolly mammoths. Thirdly, I was a 'specky four-eyes', and my hair had a habit of sticking out at angles, and all attempts to look neat and sophisticated were somehow reversed on the school bus. The rest just rolled into place.

It was further accommodated by a bullying teacher who delighted in mocking children so that she could get laughs from the rest of the class. Some of the worst school stories I have heard from people are when it was a teacher who started the bullying. Looking back, there are few things I find more pathetic than the teacher who curries favour with the majority of their class by picking on the othered children, just like that cheap hack comic having a go at 'that fat man

WEIRDO or WHEN DID YOU REALIZE YOU WERE ODD?

in the front row' or 'you with the horrible shirt you're wearing for a bet'. Forty years on, I met someone I was at school with. We had a drink, and our conversation soon turned to the French teacher who had picked on him so much you could still see the damage.

I forced myself into ways of trying to fit in. I learned how to adopt the pose of paying attention. I learned that I couldn't play sport and the more aware I became of that, the worse I was at it. The more I tried, the more I failed. So I avoided it wherever I could. I was banned from using an ink pen as I was able to distribute ink almost everywhere but on the page.

It was also at school that I learned some useful skills that have helped my work and adult life. I am adept at procrastinating, but when the steel teeth of a deadline start to bite deeply, I will rise to the occasion. My weekend homework was always done on Sunday night covertly under the blankets. Though often ill-prepared for essays and exams, when my chaotic mind was forced to focus, I could achieve good grades and even occasionally win prizes. It is something I still rely on today. A racing mind can be poor for classroom etiquette and general coherence but can perform wonders in a tense situation of 'turn over your papers, two hours, starting NOW!' Who is that annoying child who has asked for more paper? ME! I did not approach exams confidently. I had never revised enough as words didn't seem to go in. But then this strange splurge of connections would occur for a couple of hours, a manic eruption of ideas.

For ASD pupils, taking exams can be particularly stressful, starting with the question of understanding why they need to do an exam to prove their ability in the first place. Exams can create high anxiety for those ASD pupils who find it difficult to adjust to new and unusual experiences and settings. And the very phrasing of exam questions can also be confusing. Quite rightly, there are now guidelines asking exam boards to very carefully think about how their questions and papers are structured so that those with ASD aren't hamstrung before even opening the exam paper.

NORMALLY WEIRD AND WEIRDLY NORMAL

Boarding school

The real impact of school hit me when I was thirteen and sent to boarding school. Here the loneliness was intense because there was nowhere to be alone, nowhere to hide, unless you had measles, and sadly I had already had measles so there was no infirmary retreat for me. This was when the loneliness of unwanted company crushed all possibility of the happiness of solitude. There was always someone around the corner hoping to catch you out or belittle you, often in the hope of taking the heat off their own situation for a while. It was an oppressive cocktail of dormitory tribalism and puberty – the worst of times. Boarding school is a place where conformity is essential, a training ground designed to lead men to death in war or be prime management material in the tobacco industry.

I liked to be solitary. I liked to read alone. I liked movies about Frankenstein and werewolves, and I liked pondering witchcraft and demonology. I was not socially rambunctious. I found conversations hard to join in with because everyone, as far as I was concerned, seemed to be interested in the same boring things I wasn't interested in. I could not find common ground with anyone. I was both continually anxious and bored. I could not find anywhere or anyone that fitted me. I would spend a lot of my time daydreaming about suicide.

I was not a noisy rebel, but at the same time, I couldn't seem to find a way to be correctly institutionalized. My skull would echo with a thousand whys. I felt a total outsider in an institution that was meant to make insiders, meant to bind us together by our school motto and our school ties, readying us for the S&M dungeon of business, politics and high finance.

WEIRDO or WHEN DID YOU REALIZE YOU WERE ODD?

Letters home

My eldest sister recently found all the letters that I sent to my mum from school. She wondered why my parents didn't take me out. I thought I'd covered up what I felt most of the time, but she read between the lines of my letters and saw the quiet desperation there. I thought I was doing a wizard job of concealment, but it turns out I was not so adept at masking everything.

The letter that I remember most was a letter my sister could never read – the first letter I sent home, before my acts of concealment, when my desperation was at its loudest and most raw. I begged to come home and promised that I would sell my books or toys or whatever was needed to start paying back that term's fees. Sadly for me, the letter was first found in my desk by another boy at the school, snooping around for weakness and weapons of mockery. It gave the 'in-crowd' more ammo and gave me more shame. I sent it, but that first Christmas, when I came home for the holiday, I found the bedside cupboard where my mum kept the letters, removed that one and ripped it to pieces before setting fire to it. I was letting people down and I had to cover the tracks of my feelings.

Looking through the letters that remain, I see the common theme is boredom and, at times, some honesty about my experience. But the honesty diminishes with each term as I learned to mask my inner life.

> *I am being teased in class, sometimes in English and History as they are my best subjects . . . can I come out one Sunday before half term, in about 3 weeks time, as all the other boys go out sometimes?*

I can visualize that boy and feel his feelings, and I know how alone he was and how desperate he was to get that little escape.

NORMALLY WEIRD AND WEIRDLY NORMAL

So far, I've earned the name Gutsy from a prefect called Judd.

I added his height of '6 foot 5' for some reason. Although nothing ever happened, he always made me stay longer in the communal showers after games which I was slightly suspicious of and unnerved by. I was called Gutsy because I had puppy fat.* Indeed, I viewed myself as considerably fatter than I was from quite an early age. I am surprised by images of my teenage self because I look so much thinner than the wobbly thing I imagined I was. I saw myself as the poster outside a circus sideshow in Alabama, while I was really little more than a beaming boy in a 1950s advert for porridge oats.

PE is impossible. Circuit training every week.

I signed off with a note of happiness.

I loved John Wyndham and had taken my big book of John Wyndham to school, so I was delighted that one of the first books we studied was *The Chrysalids*, a book that resonated particularly with me as I was increasingly identifying as a chrysalid myself. The chrysalids of the story are those people with mutations, sometimes very negligible ones, but however marginal the mutation they are banished and considered a blasphemy. I had very small thumbs (I still do) and, for the first few terms, I developed a lazy R when I spoke, all of which added to the feeling of being different, an outsider . . . a chrysalid.

A few weeks later, I wrote home again.

I hope everything is well, we have been doing very little at the moment except our cleaning duties and things. Life isn't too bad, but I'm not enjoying it that much as everyone in my year is teasing and bullying me.

* Now it is merely middle-age fat, but I did have a brief period of being skinny.

WEIRDO or WHEN DID YOU REALIZE YOU WERE ODD?

Seeing these letters for the first time in forty years, I was surprised by my honesty, and it tells me, for me to have revealed anything, I must have hated it with a vengeance. I soon move on to hoping my mum found what she wanted when she went to St Albans, probably a headscarf and woollen jumper, before writing about elephants.

> *Have you read in the papers about Pole, the elephant Bill Travers and Virginia McKenna are trying to get taken back to Africa because of its lonely conditions in London Zoo.*

I don't think it was intentional, but I read that now and wonder whether I was really saying, 'I wonder if Bill Travers and Virginia McKenna could campaign to get me out of *this* zoo as my condition is lonely too.'

I couldn't get anything right. In that first year, I made friends with a boy called Giles. I stayed with him for a few days during the summer holiday and his two cats kept the family awake by having that agonizing howling sex that cats seem to have. When we were back at school, I told the story of the cats, just thinking it was silly and would allow me to do the spot-on howling cat sex noise I had perfected. And that was that – end of friendship. He saw my recounting as ridicule, but it really wasn't. I was not trying to gain power by belittling his noisy sex cats. I didn't understand it. The only ones embarrassed should have been the cats, but apparently, feline shame is impossible. I was not good at treading through the politics; I remained naive. I still find myself saying things which I think are quite socially acceptable or fun then being told I have very much misjudged things.

For some boys, there were mental and physical reactions to the stress of boarding school. One thirteen-year-old boy lost all his hair to alopecia; another took to walking three steps forward and two steps back wherever he went, as if escaping from the rules of walking forward meant he was escaping a little bit from the world.

NORMALLY WEIRD AND WEIRDLY NORMAL

I tried to keep my head down, but not so far down that it made it easier to shove it in the toilet bowl.

Weakness, bullying and resilience

An early reader pointed out that I had written about how I was picked on for being weak, but not about how it felt to be weird. They asked me if I could explain how I was weird, how I experienced that otherness.

And here lies a problem that I think is illustrative. I was not a cyclops, I did not have the ears of a mule, I did not break into arias from *La Traviata* or the chorus of Gary Numan's 'Cars' in the middle of geography. I was just me, with a head full of anxiety, fear and babbling thoughts that I was keeping in successfully, most of the time. It is the 'weirdness' on the inside, not what makes you odd on the exterior that can make school a battleground. It is something that detaches you and others you, and that's what your peers pick up on. I think it comes down to a total lack of any sense of connection with other people, a feeling that there are things wrong with your thoughts and also your flesh, an innate sense of being a pariah. That is the best I can do.

I asked Charlie, an old friend from school, who is now a popular teacher in a comprehensive school, what he remembers of being on the outside in the inside world of public school. He feels like we refused to compromise on being anything but ourselves, which made things more difficult, but ultimately, it meant we left with our personalities intact and undiluted by compromise and cognitive dissonance.

Charlie also had a lot of hidden trauma, which helped his defiance. He would explode with anger at times and once, very effectively, punched Adam Thomas for saying that his girlfriend 'must be a munter because you are too'. That was the last time Adam Thomas insulted Charlie, perhaps discovering he was not so 'weak' after all. Charlie thinks our experience of trauma from before boarding

WEIRDO or WHEN DID YOU REALIZE YOU WERE ODD?

school coloured us, and actually 'gave us a steel that maybe others didn't have'. Though we were not unscathed during our time there, perhaps we were less damaged by the experience than some of those who appeared to thrive. I am glad to say that he remembers me being 'very funny' which probably helped propel the punches in my direction because 'no one likes a smart-arse'. Though, actually, some people do like a smart-arse, especially if they are getting the better of a dumb-arse with a bullying habit. It's worth the bloody nose, a wound of victory.

I have found many people, who now consider themselves neurodivergent, find compromise very difficult if it means compromising their sense of fairness or compromising their sense of self. To obey when it clashes with your ethics is disturbing and can lead to many issues at school or work. 'Why don't you just do what you're told?' There is a tenacity and a refusal to back down, even when it would be advantageous, because it just isn't right.

I feel like I walked away without being shaped by the system as it intended, and that, in the long term, was far better for me than for many of those around me. What I learned from the system was that many things about it were wrong and that there were many other examples of flawed systems throughout the world.

In the final year, I experienced a strange sort of victory. The resilience paid off, and with it, there came a grudging respect from others. In failing to be truly crushed or reshaped, and with 'release' imminent, I went from being a victim to a 'character'. It was like a mini version of the first time I played the Belfast Empire. I was booed throughout my set and had things thrown at me, but I didn't leave early, and so everyone wanted to buy me a pint afterwards, both loathed and admired . . . and eventually inebriated.

My closest friend at boarding school was my pal Ed. I think we saw through the nonsense of speeches from the headmaster about us being 'the best of Britain' quite early on. Our friendship started strongly. The first time I spoke to him, he told me to 'piss off'. We were on a school coach back from rowing training and his face was purple from the exertion. I said something good-natured about it being a horrible and sweaty experience and, having been at school for two terms now, Ed presumed I must have been taking the mickey out of him, because that is what everyone did. That was the currency. This is where the tedium of 'banter' takes hold. The idea that someone was just being friendly with no agenda had already been made totally alien. The fragility of these boys meant friendships could be utterly destroyed by any incident that was perceived as threatening your psychological survival.

However, unlike my cat sex impressions, this was not the end of all possibilities. Fortunately, Ed and I later bonded over a copy of *Starburst* magazine, a magazine covering films of the fantastical. This issue had Leonard Nimoy on the cover. We had a long time to talk about the magazine because, for most of those sports lessons, it was decided by everyone that it would be best if Ed and I stood by the wall, off the pitch, so as not to cause a sporting failure.

I had already realized the world was going to be a difficult fit for me, but Ed arrived in this new world of ours without such baggage. When I asked him recently how he felt now about those school years, he was forthright.

> *'I disliked almost everything about it. I'm fifty-four now; I've lived through my dad getting Alzheimer's and dying of COVID, my mum getting Parkinson's and dying of sepsis, my sister's battles with both alcoholism and severe mental health issues, along with my own ups and downs, of course. Yet those five years at that school remain unquestionably the worst period in my life. They took a happy and confident thirteen-year-old and turned him into a chronically under-confident eighteen-year-old.'*

Listening to this both broke my heart and brought it all back.

Public school is a good model of how the status quo of society as a

WEIRDO or WHEN DID YOU REALIZE YOU WERE ODD?

whole works, of how bullying is a central plank in society's structure, of how anyone who steps out of line or is unable to toe such a line becomes marked, of how privilege is currency and how obedience is deemed essential if you want to be part of it all. This was something Lindsay Anderson's celebrated film *If . . .* dealt with. The location he used for his public school that represented empire and eventual revolution was his old school, Cheltenham College, which was where Ed and I experienced our archaic education too. Anderson's critique was so accurate that he was banned from returning to the school for some years. Over the years, there has been some solace for me in watching Malcolm McDowell mowing down the staffroom with a machine gun from the roof of the building where we learned about glacial valleys and the English Civil War. My education was meant to make me loyal to King and Country, though I think it actually strengthened my republicanism and my scepticism about national pride.

The best thing that came out of my school experience was a lifelong friendship with Ed. Ed would not describe himself as neurodivergent, though that chronic lack of confidence that was thrust upon him is certainly something shared with many neurodivergent people. But your weirdness does not need to be diagnosable; weird can just be not genuflecting to the system. He explained that, for decades afterwards, he was completely unaware that he never looked anyone in the eye in conversation, and remained convinced, deep down, that he was ugly and unappealing. He instinctively looked for and expected the worst in people and in the wider world, because the worst had shown up so often at school. He remembered those boys who would casually wander into the dormitory to see who didn't fit in, to see if they could be made to fit in even less. The bullying boys who would sit bare-arsed and unwiped on younger boys' faces if the taunting and mockery wasn't giving them enough kicks. He remembers that the boys in his own year stripped him naked, then dragged him 'down the cold, tiled boarding house corridor at night, then held me down while one dripped hot wax onto my genitals'. What the system deemed character-building was character-destroying.

I think much of what we camouflage as character-building in the world is actually destructive and aimed towards generating a culture of compliance. Some boys changed their personalities to fit in, so they could ally themselves with the bullies. They were masking, but some didn't just mask, they cut off their old face and made a nasty new one.

One day, Ed's housemaster, who for some reason had the nickname 'Pissy Willy', shouted in an annoyed manner that Ed's mother and father were on the phone, making much of this personal inconvenience to him. The housemaster knew what the phone call was about, Ed did not.

Ed's grandmother had died.

Such lack of compassion is part of a system which makes compassion and empathy a weakness. Looking back, Ed says:

'That's probably what I disliked the most: the completely warped sense of life that it gave me, and the years it took to fully understand that the world is not this way, and neither am I. It's a place filled with love, joy, laughter and compassion.'

Later, in the lower sixth, girls joined the school. Similar 'normality' was on display here. Any boy who behaved as if girls were normal humans you could talk to was seen as suspect and ridiculous. Misogyny was rife, in both the sixth form common room and the staff room. Charlie remembered that, if you sat and talked to girls, then 'the usual suspects' would come and dump spoons on the table, to symbolize your status as 'spooners'.* He also recalled the day a

---

* An undoubtedly derogatory term – I had no idea then, or even now, what it meant, but by God, the pathetic-ness of it all bites hard even today.

WEIRDO or WHEN DID YOU REALIZE YOU WERE ODD?

teacher told one of the girls to make him a cup of tea. She was fortunate enough to find some curdled milk and ensured she created the most disgusting tea possible.

Ed and I were lucky. We left the institution still believing that this normal was not a good or a right normal. Sadly, much of wider society still abides by the rules we experienced. Charlie met up with some old classmates and found that one former bully was filled with guilt and regret. Their abusive behaviour had come from their own struggles, another casualty of the world of concealment. There was one boy who struggled more than the others. Like Ed, when I first tried to be friendly, he lashed out. At thirteen years old, he just wanted to keep playing with his toy cars, so he was relentlessly abused. He became unreachable. Looking back now, I think it is highly likely that he was neurodivergent. A few of us have tried to find out his whereabouts, but with no success. He has vanished. Some fear he may have taken his own life.

Charlie muses on his working life now and says:

'Working at a comprehensive, it seems healthily normal. There are still groups, as in there are the awkward, slightly introvert ones, the defiantly themselves group, the "cool" groups, the dicks, but in the comprehensive environment and with this generation being more open-minded, they all tolerate each other. And I think my experience means I nip the slightest sniff of bullying in the bud.'

Other people's stories

I asked a wide group of neurodivergent people when it was in their lives that they realized those on the outside thought they were weird, and 'at school' was frequently given as the answer, the environment where, like Ed, their happiness was stripped from them because they weren't 'right'. It can come as a rude awakening to realize others think you are weird, followed by a sharp increase in anxiety and a vast amount of energy being used to conceal your true self. Every time you are too tired to keep up the wall, the hordes rush in.

Lizzie, who I first met at university when she was a goth and when I had a quiff as high as the sky, says that she knew she was weird at nursery school. She thinks at that point it worked in her favour, but then she remembers secondary school. 'Oh dear God, that was *awful*. Suddenly, being weird engendered a tidal wave of ridicule balanced beautifully by social exclusion.'

She was fortunate to have a dad who reassured her that 'all the narrow-minded sheep-folk would be weeded out once I went to college'. Fortunately, this proved to be right. 'I stayed weird, but so did a significant proportion of my newly found peers who had survived other secondary schools just like mine, with similar stories to share.'

Mabel thinks that primary school was where she started to feel the interrogating gaze of other people. She says that, within about a year of starting school, other kids didn't want to play with her, and teachers were always telling her off even when she got the answers right. She was told off for having too much imagination, for daydreaming, for stammering, for being clumsy, for crying too much or for being too happy. It was actually her teachers who coined her first bullying nickname and kids sang it while dancing round her in circles.

Some can conceal their feelings, often at great emotional cost, while others find this concealing act impossible to carry off. At school, Mabel would get very engaged and excited by stories or information but then discovered slowly that being excited and showing it was the wrong attitude, but even then, she found it difficult to conceal her genuine feelings just for the sake of conforming.

Octavia discovered that such behaviour was still classified as wrong when she was training as a therapist. She was described as being 'uncontained'.

WEIRDO or WHEN DID YOU REALIZE YOU WERE ODD?

'I would interrupt and get excited. I mean, that was so shameful. I remember once that the tutor shushed me. I put my hand on my mouth and tears came to my eyes. And then I realized I had bright red lipstick on, and I had smeared it wildly with my hand. So then I was trying to see what I looked like and it was What Ever Happened to Baby Jane.*'*

Look at our world and look at our news media and you see how much of it is critical, condescending and joyless – we see that in our society too. Some days on the train, being unable to mute other people's conversations, I collate them in my head instead and then build a mind graph of their content. Sadly, the disgruntled and the dismissive nearly always outweigh the excited and loving conversations.

After a gig, I was at the theatre bar with Jeevi, who makes a lot of neurodiverse TikTok content, and her autistic husband, who happened to be wearing a T-shirt for a band I am keen on, 65daysofstatic. Straight away we were talking excitedly about music, art, science and brains. Halfway through our conversation, Jeevi said that she was quite used to people hearing her excitement and having a 'yeah whatever' response. I don't want to live in a 'yeah whatever' world, in a world that roots out non-conformity and brands it as weirdness and weakness, where expressions of passion can make you weird. How weird is that?

Mabel's school brought in an educational psychologist to assess her in year 5 and didn't tell her mum it was happening. She is now a teacher herself and said she will always be shocked that they kept the assessment from her mum and also didn't clock that her mind was ASD or ADHD. She was labelled as 'severely emotionally disturbed' and then they told her mother it was because she was a single parent. Her mother reported it and eventually got a letter of apology from the council. The school was told to apologize but never did.

NORMALLY WEIRD AND WEIRDLY NORMAL

Holly was the neurodivergent child of neurodivergent parents, so she, too, only found out what normal was supposed to be when she went to school.

Stefania said her mother confessed that she started finding her 'weird' when she was about nine months old and began to speak.

Dunja, an accomplished violinist at an early age, remembers her childhood as a lovely cocktail of being called a 'wonder child' but then having the weirdest level of self-awareness, of being bullied for being weird and 'just generally feeling like an alien' because her own view of the world and her feelings did not match those around her. She has been interrogating herself and researching who she is for as long as she can remember.

Some were marked out as 'the bad seed' with no knowledge of what made them a plague carrier to other children and adults.

Maria said she was about eight when a girl at school, who she was desperately trying to be friends with, told her that her mum had instructed her to keep away from her because she was weird. Playtime was lonely for her, so she joined clubs where you didn't have to endure the bullying or solitude. Crochet club, chess club, drama club, recorder club, all met after school, but you could also stay indoors at break time for practice. Fifty years later, she is still a serial collector of hobbies.

Jojo remembers overhearing the parents of one of her friends discussing her like she was some kind of disease. Throughout childhood, up until she moved to London at seventeen, she was always described as being a bad influence on her friends, despite being pretty much scared of her own shadow because of the regular beatings her mother dished out. JoJo recently realized her mother was undiagnosed, with possibly autism or maybe ADHD, and she saw traits in her daughter she could not bear, as they both held a mirror up to her and possibly brought out the fear of a life repeated, so she tried to beat it out of her.

In so many of the stories I heard, almost no one had a memory of

WEIRDO OR WHEN DID YOU REALIZE YOU WERE ODD?

a particular action or statement that made them weird – they just carried weirdness with them. It was almost as if they began to notice that they were not aerodynamic when they tried to swim through the world, and that the lifeguards often didn't like the look of them and certainly wouldn't come to their aid. It was sink or swim.

Does the system really fall apart if the lines are not so straight? Do we look at a society that has been so healthy for so long with such fear that we see a little elasticity as such a threat? It seems to me that the weakness is not in the weirdos, but in a society that is so scared of difference that people have to mark out those who are different and harass them. I like dandelions but would love to see more orchids in the garden.

In my audiences, there are often teenagers who I know are likely to feel they will never find their place, and I make a point of talking about how school can seem like the whole world for ever, but I hope they will find their people, even if it might not be until they leave the schoolyard for the final time.

But we are not weird – it's just that they are too normal. And some of them don't even want to be normal, they just haven't found their way out. This is where the work in memory of Sophie Lancaster is so important, not merely helping the kids who are obviously different from the outside to be understood but to also show the kids who might think they have to be 'normal' that there are other possibilities of how they can be.

Sophie's mother, Sylvia, described the aims of her work as: 'to get out there and raise awareness. Let young people see that there's nothing to be frightened of, that we should be embracing difference, not scared of it'. Or as autistic actor Chloé Hayden reminds us, to be different is not to be less. Rather than the weirdos being weak, the ridicule and the bullying really come from the weakness of those who feel threatened by difference.

3. FRIENDSHIP

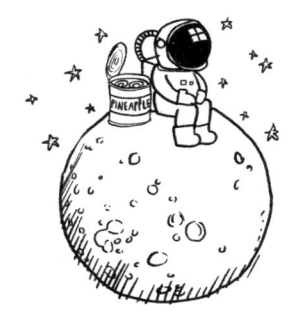

Have you got a 'best friend'?
   Have you got enough friends?
   Do you have too many friends?
   Do you not like your friends?
   Are you happy just to be alone?

Friends are apparently a necessity for survival in our society in much the same way as emoticons and nail bars. Human beings are societal creatures, so people who are just happy in their own company may be viewed with suspicion and seen as a bit 'weird'. For many people though, friends form the most influential relationships of their lives. But like other aspects of living in a communal society, there are many rules of friendship, and navigating them can often be more difficult for neurodivergent people.

My favourite fantasy as a child was to be alone. I wanted to be Robinson Crusoe. While everyone else was playing cowboys and arguing over who was going to be Wild Bill Hickok, I would want to go off to the woods alone to hide from cannibals and shadowy phantasms or to work on the coconut-inspired interior design of my cave. I could be an isolated spaceman marooned on an alien planet in an escape pod. I could imagine the dream crater where my pod would lie, peeking out from the extraterrestrial quicksand, snug but well equipped, with a kitchenette and plenty of tinned pineapple. I wanted to seek and explore a mysterious imaginary landscape.

My imagination was more 'action rambling through an extraterrestrial landscape' than 'laser gun feuds' – more botany than battle. I was always more interested in the catering facilities than the killing. I wish I still had the drawings I did every Friday night when I was allowed to have my tea watching Sherlock Holmes movies on the telly. I would draw the same giant underground mining machine, filling it with friendly machines and lounge areas. When I chose a bicycle, while all other boys had Choppers or Grifters for speed and wheelies, I chose the Raleigh Traveller for adventures, with ginger beer and ham-and-turkey sandwiches.

Being alone

I had an Action Man, the boy's Barbie with an interest in combat rather than compact mirrors. He wasn't a team player either. When my grandmother took me to the toyshop in Little Chalfont for my birthday treat, rather than choosing a soldier or a sailor, I chose the one in chunky knitwear who climbed alone. He was the nearest you could get to a birdwatcher.

'What's your Action Man doing?'

'Mine's fighting at the Battle of Monte Cassino in his big tank.'

'Mine's snorkelling with a bomb in his hand to sink a U-boat.'

'Mine's protecting a puffin's nest on Lundy Island and hoping to go to Nepal to write poetry in isolation.'

Had there been a pacifist Action Man whose gripping hands clasped Bertrand Russell's *The Problems of Philosophy*, I would probably have chosen him.

During my childhood, I got hold of a couple more Action Men, but my Action Man needed no company. I would just strip them for parts. My original Action Man did not have proper gripping hands, so I gave him a hand transplant. Then, with the new ones, I would

FRIENDSHIP

see what happened if you held them over an open fire and melted them down or shaved their beards. How would his face drip?

Looking back, I don't think playing alone made me sad. I think I enjoyed it. It was just that everyone else thought I needed company. There was a time when I wanted to be popular, but I think that was for the achievement of being popular, rather than what you truly gained from friendship. This didn't mean I didn't want friends, but I think, at times, I wanted to have friends because I knew you were meant to have friends. Adults can't believe a child can want to be solitary. 'There's a boy your age down the street. You can be friends.' Being alone is translated as being unhappy. Surely hanging out in a gang is happier.

But with companionship come hierarchies and competitiveness, and I just wasn't very good at 'boy' boy things. I tried. I once bought a football magazine and a book to put stickers of football players in, but my heart wasn't really in it. I was pretending to be a boy.

The general rule was that I would eventually be friendly with the last three boys who were standing by the fence as the football teams were being picked (by the time I got to know Ed, I was older and so that is why we were standing by a wall). Our wheezy ineptitude meant we were chosen not for our skills, which were non-existent, but for who carried the lowest risk of getting in the way. And the less you tried, the better. The try-hard would always end up tripping over and landing in front of your own centre forward just as he was about to shoot and score.

But the wider social pressure of being seen to have friends meant I invited far too many people to my tenth birthday party. Michael Cunliffe removed all the sweets from my piece of birthday cake when I had to leave the room to talk to Uncle Hans on the phone, and when I returned, everyone laughed at me and my desecrated cake, while Michael Cunliffe sat hamster-cheeked, full to the brim with candies.

Being comfortable alone brings on suspicion. But pretending to be what you are not can be agonizing. At boarding school, one of my secret places of retreat was late-night radio. For me, it was an exotic place of alternative voices and strange music. It was on those wavelengths that I discovered the Scottish poet Ivor Cutler on the *John Peel Show* and he shared a striking piece of advice on how to make a friend. Cutler advised knocking an open pot of paint off a windowsill onto a random passer-by. Then you should invite the furious bespattered person up to your flat to get clean. Once they were in the bath, you should inspect their clothes for holes, and if you noticed a hole in their vest, you should mend it for them. Though he stated that the choice of thread was yours, he preferred tailor's thread because every time their skin was irritated by the thread, it would be a memory of your friendship.

For many people, school is where long-lasting friendships are forged. There are people who leap at the chance of school reunions, people who are married to people they first met at school, social groups that are still based on all being in the same school rugby team, a bond made even stronger if all fifteen were in a remote plane crash followed by survival cannibalism in their graduation year.

For others, it is only after escaping the rigorous social repetition of school when possibilities of true friendship can begin. Freed from the wrought-iron fencing of the school fields, I felt a rapid depressurization during my journey to the surface and the sunlight. Would I now find 'my people'? And if so, who would they be?

Rejection!

Though I would have liked to have had a girlfriend, I had no belief that I would ever have one and was quite sure that this would always be the case. With both friendship and romantic possibilities, humans fear rejection.

We can all be preoccupied with rejection, even with a brain where the prefrontal cortex and executive function is firing roughly as

FRIENDSHIP

intended. How much do we miss out on because 'what could have been' is an easier daydream than risking the failure of what was right there in front of us? To risk rejection is to risk shattering your dream.

Like so much on the neurodiversity spectrum, while everyone has probably experienced such inertia, there is a point on the dial where rejection anxiety becomes overwhelmingly dominant. For both autistic and ADHD people, there is a heightened sensitivity to perceived rejection, a sensitivity that means you can experience all the negatives of rejection based on the slightest of hunches, the smallest of facial gestures, the tone of a single syllable. It's known in the psychology business as rejection sensitive dysphoria (RSD). It can be experienced by people with anxiety and a strong desire for validation. This can mean that both making friends and keeping friends is very difficult. Both the fear and reality of rejection can be physically sickening.

If you have built-in low self-esteem, it seems natural to think, 'Why would this person want to be friends with me?' or to presume the only reason they are maintaining a friendship is not because they like you but because you are useful in some way.

'It must be because I drive a car and can give them lifts.'

'It must be because they like my sister.'

'It must be because I look like someone who would be tasty if we were in a plane crash together.'

When I consider my own group of friends, I seem to have collected one from each period of my life: one from school, one from my first job, one from university, one from my second job, and then a sort of loose collective from all the decades of my peripatetic life of showing off. Despite the length of time I have been friends with this limited group – three of them for over thirty years – it is only in the past two years or so that I have lost my anxiety in their company. The same commentary would run through me.

Before I met up with them, I would have pre-gig nerves. 'What if

I can't think of anything to say?' Then, it would begin.

'Was I wrong to hug them?'

'Are they annoyed I didn't hug them?'

'Am I boring them?'

'Am I talking too much?'

'Do I look like I am showing off?'

'Would they prefer it if I was not here?'

'Have the *me* conversations far outnumbered the *them* conversations?'

And so on.

As someone who knows how terrifying fearing rejection or disdain can be, I have found systems based on openness and honesty which I can adopt when talking to other people that I hope reduce their fears. After my shows, I am usually accessible, whether stood by a merchandise table or in the bar. People often want to know how stories that got derailed by tangents actually ended or want to share an experience that they have been reminded of by the show. Sometimes, people tell me funny stories, and sometimes, there are sad stories of loss. I can sometimes see in people's faces, mid-story, that they may be beginning to think, *Why am I telling this stranger my story? He must be bored or embarrassed. I bet he has something better to do and can't wait for me to finish.*

Well, I rarely have better things to do after a show beyond returning to my inauspicious hotel. I believe it is a great privilege for people to trust you so much that they are prepared to share their lives with you. So before they depart, I now have a habit of openly saying, 'Just in case you are worried, because I know in similar situations I have left the room and immediately started analysing why I said all I said and berating myself and overthinking, I want you to know that I am glad you took time to talk to me and happy that you felt you could tell me your story.' It might not entirely stem their post-conversation paranoia, but hopefully, it is a start.

One of the reasons I have wanted to bring ideas like this into

FRIENDSHIP

the sunlight was made manifest at a book festival gig on the edge of Reading. While I was signing books, the mother of the festival organizer came up to me. I had been talking about the critical voice that won't shut up, that tells us everything we are saying is being received politely but that our friends really think we are idiotic. She had not known other people experienced this. She thought it was just her. She was in her seventies and had not known that the oppressive, negative, critical voice she heard inside her head was in other people's heads too. She seemed genuinely surprised and, I think, a little relieved too. I was glad.

The rules of friendship

There are unwritten rules of how friendships work. Gatherings of friends will include banter, nicknames and burnt-meat barbecues if it is sunny. There is regularity and a pattern, codes of matey-ness that can seem inscrutable to anyone on the outside, let alone those whose patterns of thought and social perception are so different.

Perhaps it would be best to define friendship through academic research. The conceptual definition, based on the work of Bauminger, Solomon, Aviezer, Heung, Gazit, et al. is 'stable, frequent, and interconnected affective interactions that are manifested by certain classes of behavioural markers (e.g., sharing, play and conversational skills) that facilitate the functions of companionships, intimacy, and closeness'.[1] This was the starting point when studying childhood friendship patterns with ASD kids.

Research demonstrated that children and adolescents with ASD had fewer friends than their neurotypical peers. One in five ASD young people believe they have no friends at all, and those who believe they have at least one friend experience friendships with shorter durations than neurotypical young people. In the *Encyclopedia of Autism Spectrum Disorders*, the entry on understanding friendships states that children and adolescents with

ASD reported 'lower levels of companionship, security-intimacy, closeness and help than their matched typically developing peers, with the majority of differences reaching significance'.[2] The quality of friendship also declined as the children got older, while conflict increased.

In 'Setbacks and Success: How Young Adults on the Autism Spectrum Seek Friendship', the researchers concluded that 'friendship for people on the autism spectrum is lacking when compared with their typically developing peers'.[3] It might also be a story of difference rather than deficit. 'From this and other studies, it is clear that people on the autism spectrum may perceive friendship differently, have different priorities or goals for friendship, and have different ways of seeking and experiencing friendship than their typical peers.'

I have certainly found it common that the expectations of friendship are different among many neurodivergent people. I have always found it hard to define who my friends are, as if putting the title of friend on them places far too great a pressure and expectation while also creating a certainty. I am not good with certainties and worry far too much about expectations.

When I spoke to the naturalist and campaigner Chris Packham about how he had experienced the years before he was diagnosed as autistic, he told me that, during his university years, he had no friends. This was not because he was rejected by others, but because he rejected the idea of having friends. He felt that friendship would get in the way of him getting the biology degree he so wanted. He told me this didn't mean he didn't talk to anyone, but he summed up his interactions with others as, 'Get out of the way, I want to get into this lecture.' Now he has friends, but they are very specific to what he needs. He has someone to talk to about birds, someone to talk to about punk rock, and so on. It seems like a good system to me.

For some ASD people, friendships can be more difficult because of the difficulty of understanding social cues and non-verbal

FRIENDSHIP

communication, which, with the addition of social anxiety, can make experiences overwhelming. Take so-called 'banter'. Banter is a popular way among friends of having fun, mocking your friends' weight, partners, debatable sexuality, haircuts, football teams, etc. Backstage at comedy clubs is often vibrant with putdowns and gallows humour about your performance.

Banter can be fear-inducing, raising anxiety and apprehension, and for those with ASD, there's a great difficulty in working out exactly what is amusing 'banter' and what is really speaking to truth. My need to banter has declined as my understanding of my mind and my perception of the inner lives of others has increased. My experience in conversations with neurodivergent people is that, while there can be plenty of jokes, there is very little banter, not so many instances where someone in the group is the butt of such laughter. I think that with many neurodivergent people's experience of being bullied, taunted or ostracized, there can be a far greater sensitivity to such humour and a sensitivity towards the feelings of others. I've found this frees people to be more open and more fun because you're not constantly on edge, waiting to find out if they're next. Much like the comedians who say jokes can't exist without a victim for a punchline, I think the idea that socializing can't be fun without taking the piss just shows a lack of effort and imagination.

Jamie Knight is ASD and an active campaigner for disability rights. He has a tremendous awareness of the stumbling blocks that come with neurodivergence in many different spheres. One of his activities has been group sessions with people who believe they are socially awkward and as a result saw themselves as terrible and incapable people. During the gentle coaching sessions, everyone gets a chance to know each other and talk more, and often the conclusion that Jamie and others come to is that actually the problem wasn't with them, it was just that certain of their friends 'were assholes'.

Perhaps this is where others might find it all a bit odd, the amount of thought that goes into the very nature of friendship and what a friend may be. Such overthinking can be crippling but it can also be very rewarding. Once you start to understand your 'algorithm' for the way your friendships work, what you need from a friendship, then the fog can lift and friendships can strengthen, though some may fall away. It becomes important to know that your people are out there.

Love means never having to say, 'Sorry, who are you again?'

Joanna Neary is a comedian, writer and artist (self-portrait below). Joanna and her family have found life together much easier since they found a new context for her behaviour. She is late-diagnosed ADHD, with the added possibility of being on the autistic spectrum. When she wasn't with her family physically, Joanna struggled at times to keep in mind even those who she loved most deeply. This is called object permanence and is related to inattention and is often an issue for ADHD people when things or people are literally 'out of sight, out of mind'. People with ADHD typically may lose objects they need, forget about tasks . . . or forget about their husband.

Joanna's husband used to get quite upset by her behaviour. He found it very disconcerting that Joanna could go away and not miss him at all. Absence, after all, is meant to make the heart grow fonder, not make the brain forget you exist. Not long after they first became a couple, she went away for a month to perform at the Edinburgh Fringe Festival. Her husband would call to say how much he missed her. Joanna would distractedly reply, 'Okay. Right . . .' He didn't understand why she didn't say she missed him too. Surely, she should be lovelorn and pining for him, like he was for her. He started to worry that she was going to run off with someone else. As Joanna told me, it probably didn't help

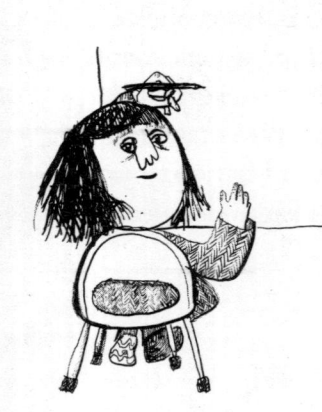

FRIENDSHIP

that she'd told him a number of stories about how actors and directors had flings when on tour, just before she departed. But now he knows that her detachment from him when she is away is just the way her mind works.

The heartstrings are detachable when not in use, but this does not mean that they have been disposed of. She is not about to run off with someone else. In *The Articulate Autistic* blog, Jaime A. Heidel wrote about what they see as the different attitudes to friendship in autistic circles and in neurotypical groups. They define the difference using the example of cacti and roses.[4] A neurotypical friendship needs attention and maintenance, like a rose bush, while an autistic friendship is strong and unchanging and can be left alone for a while without there being any damage. I sympathize with the cactus position. It is how all my friendships work. I can go for years without contact, but the moment I get in touch again, I can pick up where I left off, sometimes almost mid-sentence. This can be tricky for people who like to feel needed and wanted.

The term 'friendship degradation mechanics' has been coined to explain this. While a neurodivergent person may see the friendship as strong, despite the lack of contact, the neurotypical person doesn't feel that way, as not enough attention has been paid, and so the friendship erodes. I like to think that neurodivergent people are less needy, but can often be very strong friends when needed. It is the pragmatic nature of the mind. When someone needs you, you will be there. There is nothing casual about the friendship, despite what others may see as its apparent infrequency. The depth of connection means that regular contact is not required. There is a naturalness to the rapport that is rekindled on contact.

I think this might also come from an honesty that people can find unsettling. I find that the banality of conversational rules is not adhered to by neurodivergents. If someone asks me how I am, I will damn well tell them how I am, and not fob them off with a dishonest 'Yeah, good thanks' if it's not the truth, and if I'm interested enough to ask the question myself, I'd expect others to do the same for me and I'd be happy to listen to their reply. As you can imagine, it is in this realm of run-of-the-mill dishonesty where connections between those perceived as neurotypical and those perceived as neurodivergent run aground.

My wife will sometimes hear me talking to a friend and look utterly perplexed by the honesty of our conversation, as well as the rapidity of our non-sequiturs and the speed of our tangents. 'Do they mind you talking like that?' she'll ask. I explain that this is just how they are talking back to me too. It is a wild ride without too many enforced niceties and rules.

The rules of 'we don't talk about that in polite society' are not adhered to. For instance, the rule that 'you should avoid talking about politics and money' seems silly to me and also helps empower the status quo. I remember being told off for directly asking how much someone's new house cost. Oh, the horror! But why is that beyond the pale? I am far happier talking about peculiar anthropological practices involving wild boar and hallucinogenic mushrooms, or the physical possibility of time loops than the latest trending series on a streaming service or some gossip about Jill and Marco, whoever they may be.

Though some may be bemused that someone is standing by the crudités considering the potential hallucinations of a hairy pig, those who are attracted to the conversation will probably be friends for life. If I socialize, and I am often asked not to, I need to feel the conversation has the possibility of thoughts that will live beyond the lounge.

But do you really need friends?

When I was talking with Octavia, she told me that she sometimes thinks, *I'll probably be alright if I never see anybody again*. And that includes her closest friends. She knows that won't happen, but she

FRIENDSHIP

says that she feels her attachment is different to a neurotypical person's attachment. When she was in training to be a therapist, she would say out loud, 'I just want this to be over,' and 'I don't really care if I never see some of these people again.' The tutors would reply, 'You can't say that!' But she could and she did.

Will society collapse if too many of us reveal what lies within and deal with each other honestly? Now in midlife, I am comfortable to be without a traditional social life because I know so many other people who are similarly comfortable with the looseness of the rules. I may not hear from pals for a very long time and they may not hear from me, but the connection between us is not broken by lack of communication.

I am happy to go alone to the cinema or to see a band. I don't know why the loner is seen as so suspicious or sad. And I am rarely alone as there is usually a book in my pocket and a couple more in my rucksack, so I always have the companionship of another person's mind and other people's stories.

I like the idea of quiet parties. There are snacks and there are drinks, and it is bring a book rather than bring a bottle. Bring a whole stack if you want. We can put them on a table in the middle of the room and people can browse through them and chat at a low level about the ones that interest them the most. Then we can all sit around in comfortable chairs and every now and again look up and say 'Ali Smith writes so beautifully about art and love' or 'Blimey, I never knew that about Sidney Poitier' – a conversation may or may not open up, and then everyone can return to reading their book and drinking their gin. The pressure to *make* conversation is removed, and we can all sit quietly until it just bubbles up.

4. THE CONVERSATION

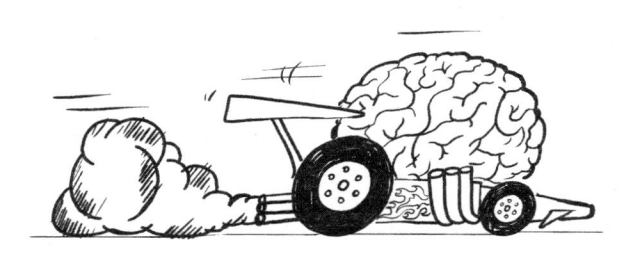

The battle for focus in racing brains

One of the first replies I received when I put out a question about how people experienced conversation was from Elizabeth, who said, 'I often have to pause in the middle of a sentence because there are so many things I could say next that I get option overload and have to start again.' I recognized the option overload moment, but rather than pausing, other responders described ploughing ahead at that instance, as I do, leaving much work for the listener who must fill in the gaps.

The theoretical physicist and mathematician Frank Wilczek believed that we probably have one billion separate thoughts during the course of our lives. This was not what he won the Nobel Prize for. He won the Nobel Prize for the 'discovery of asymptotic freedom in the theory of the strong interaction'. I would love to wax lyrical on asymptotic freedom, but sadly, due to a lack of space in this book, I will have to skip it. The best I can tell you is that 'the non-relativistic quark model simply did not make sense'. But just after I cut and pasted that I instantaneously realized I would be unable to create the illusion that I understood what I was writing about. This counts as one of my billion thoughts, with just 999,999,999 to go.

NORMALLY WEIRD AND WEIRDLY NORMAL

I am sticking with Wilczek's thought on thoughts though, because the rate of thoughts in a day is something I have often thought about (999,999,998). A common experience for neurodivergent people, particularly ADHD people, is racing thoughts. Do I squeeze in more than a billion and, if so, to what effect? A busier mind is not necessarily a better mind (999,999,997 . . . I'll stop counting there). There are some who have long, quiet periods inside their heads, but when an idea or thought pops up, it is perhaps useful or beautiful. Others don't have that many thoughts and the ones they do have are bland or ugly, and sometimes they go on with that same thought over and over again and set up a political party or get a newspaper column.

A rushing brain has its advantages. The high-speed game of cognitive tag means that thirty thoughts may be nonsensical or ludicrous or bland, but then the thirty-first thought is brilliant or invigorating. And all this has happened in under a minute or so. It's like having a brain full of typing monkeys – sure, there is a lot of blather, but some of it is really tip-top blather.

In between all the nonsense, sitting in a car on a Wolverhampton ring road, having just sung a high-pitched version of Guns N' Roses's 'Paradise City', which consisted of screeching one line over and over again (honestly, the rest of the car loved it), I suddenly had a quite brilliant idea for a film (well, I thought it was). I would make an unofficial sequel to *The Fast and the Furious* called *The Slow and the Curious*, in which we follow a bunch of petrolheads travelling at 30 miles per hour down B roads stopping at every point of interest and fragment of antiquity. Jason Statham runs all the gift shops and Vin Diesel manages a crazy golf concession in St Leonards-on-Sea.

I am sure there are many other people who generate quite a body of gibberish within their minds, but their brain presses 'delete' before it can reach their mouths. Psychologist Charles Fernyhough once told me that we should not be as worried as we often are about our thoughts because some of them are not really *our* thoughts, just

THE CONVERSATION

so much background noise, like machinery as it's clanking away. I think I probably amplify the machinery too much and see what comes of it, which is why talking to me might be as pleasurable for some as listening to Lou Reed's *Metal Machine Music*.

The sheer weight of thoughts tumbling one after the other is so great with ADHD that, if some of them aren't given an outlet, the pressure within is enough to expel ear wax at high speed and cause nosebleeds. If I don't have an outlet, then after a day or so, I will usually get a stress headache. The input and output need to be balanced to avoid aneurysms.

This thought speed is like another language. Those of us who speak it can understand it all, those who watch from the sidelines can feel as if they are caught in the maelstrom of an Esperanto discussion on fluid mechanics. When I have a beer with an ADHD pal, such as my friend Josie Long, we will rattle away into a conversational entropy filled with empathy. After three hours, we might remember where the conversation began, and aim for a dénouement, but conclusions are rare. A satisfying conclusion is not a necessity for an ADHD conversation as it is a case of the ride being more fun than the destination. There are very occasional pauses when one or other of us might say, 'Hang on, why did I bring this up?' but then we are off again into a wonderful and verdant wilderness.

When I am on stage, after ten minutes or so, members of the audience are aware they have the designated job of telling me what I started talking about and what stories I have set up before being distracted by a word that has led me down another alley. After one gig, an eighty-year-old retired builder came up to me and said, 'I didn't understand a word you were saying . . . and I've had a lovely night.' The more manically free my thoughts are, the more I can create a ride. Heckles are rare, and if they do occur, they are usually helpful, such as 'Breathe!' or 'Drink some water!'

In the early days of this book, I considered writing it as my mind works, with every tangent, cul-de-sac and racetrack, but, quite rightly perhaps, it was suggested that may not be a workable way to create a book that can be comprehended beyond being an avant-garde experiment in mind deconstruction.

If I am having a conversation with my old school friend Ed, who would describe himself as neurotypical, he is very good at saying, 'Hang on, how exactly have we got from there to here?' And that reminds me that he is an exception among my friends. And, if the breadcrumbs have not been consumed by the sparrows of my mind, I am able to retread my steps back to where it all started. It is useful to occasionally have conversations with people who can focus, especially if they know why they have to monitor you so carefully rather than merely considering you a slavering fool who has escaped from Bedlam.

Just as neurotypical people can't always understand what the hell is going on in a neurodivergent conversation, neurodivergent people often find more typical conversations frustrating. ADHD people are often surprised that people are unable to follow their train of thought or able to make the leaps of understanding that they do. My wife will often be frustrated with me when I agree to something before she has given me all the information. My racing head has leapt ahead and filled in all the details, and then gets frustrated by listening to what I believe is more information than is required. I realize this is annoying for both sides.

Other people's stories

ADHD Ruth summed it up as often being several steps ahead 'but one must be polite and allow the neurotypical to finish explaining in excruciating detail the point you got ten minutes ago!'

Julia added to that with, 'By then, you've made fifteen other connections and started a whole new conversation in your head.' Julia does not know if she is neurodivergent or 'just teetering on the edge'. She works hard on stopping interrupting herself with another

THE CONVERSATION

thought to get the point out that she wants to make but finds it exhausting, and it takes her great concentration.

If you think keeping track of an ADHDer is hard, imagine how hard it is for an ADHDer to keep track of themselves. When my act contained more jokes, I would often be unable to understand why a punchline was needed at the end of a joke, as *surely* the audience knew what I knew and didn't need the extra words to get them to the dénouement of the gag? It just seemed to be underlining what was already there.

Chris, another late-diagnosed ADHDer, told me of the relief they find when speaking to a neurodivergent friend. They see it as a time and energy saver. Chris sums it up as, 'It's like having the conversational speed limit removed.' I think this is one of the reasons so many neurodivergent people end up in neurodivergent circles long before any of them know about such things – the lack of a speed limit on thought and conversation makes them compatible.

I must be mad!

ADHD does not always look like someone jumping around like they have been fuelled by candy floss and fizzy pop, however. I have met many people who have not realized they are ADHD because they do not outwardly appear to be wild and chaotic. They just think their head is wrong, because inside their minds, it is still a ten-ring circus.

But the pressure that builds.

Even in the rarefied and privileged position I have had of predominantly working in a world with a decent amount of freedom of thought, I have felt the abrasions. For those who are bottling up and trapped in the carapace of 'normal' behaviour, their heads can be pounding and filled with vicious criticism.

I must be mad, I must be mad, I must be mad. Can they see through me? SAY NOTHING!

For those who feel caged, many have found forms of private

self-expression that may at least be a start to relieving that pressure. Writing, painting, creating, fiddling with clay, making objects and collages. I am not sure if any of my books have been completed without some reference to David Cronenberg, so here goes. His film *Scanners* is about those who can hear the thoughts of people around them, pounding away. One of those suffering has become a famous and reclusive artist. His vast, acclaimed sculptures illustrate his internal battle. Much creativity undoubtedly comes from externalizing our internal battles, but it doesn't have to be so amazing it gets to the Tate – it is enough to just get it out of you.

When I start writing, I often think of an audience member who wrote to me about how he had always thought all the dizzying abstract and surreal thoughts he had must have meant he was mad and so he should cover them up at all times. Then he discovered he was not the only one and it gave him the freedom to think about who he really was. For people like him, I imagine the whole of life was like being stoned or drunk around straight and sober people. The intense concentration that comes with having to avoid giving away any clues that you are inebriated also means you cannot have any fun, you can't just let yourself go.

Among people in both the ASD and ADHD groups, there were those who said they struggled immensely with processing what had been said to them. Donna, who is an award-winning hairdresser, said this problem of processing speech could make her job very hard. She explained, 'Sometimes it feels like the words have been said out of order, and when I ask people to repeat what they've said, it can take three attempts for me to unjumble what they've said.' She added that she felt massive internal pressure to speak and that she struggles to not interrupt and to 'behave'. Trying to hold the words in exhausts her, and she knows she says things that she really shouldn't. Like many others, she finds being herself extremely exhausting.

Even within the neurodivergent world, when ASD and ADHD

THE CONVERSATION

minds meet, problems can arise because of different styles of conversation. This was summed up by Steve, late-diagnosed with autism. He can have a problem with the speed of everyday conversation and finds processing language more difficult than many neurotypical people. He now realizes that, previously, he was relying on techniques like subconscious lip-reading. Sometimes, he will hear what he thinks is gibberish, especially if he can't watch the face of the speaker, often having to say 'Sorry?' to get people to repeat things for him, but then, during that brief window of time, his brain assigns meaning to what he heard, negating the need for the repetition. So, unless someone's speech is really clear, he would find short pauses between phrases or sentences helpful, something many ADHD people, including myself, find very difficult.

It is worth all of us thinking about how other people receive and translate our conversation and our style of speaking. If someone struggles with their hearing, it is accepted that they may ask us to speak up, although the rules of society often get in the way of this most simple of requests. Similarly, it is worth bearing in mind that we are not all operating at the same speed of comprehension. Some questions that people use in conversations, that are really just filling the gaps and are usually brushed aside with niceties, are not so simple for those with neurodivergent minds.

Bumping into an autistic pal, I fell into the traditional dull opener, 'Hello, John. How are you?' To which he replied, 'Well, that is a very complex question . . .' On this occasion, we mutually decided to move on to topic two: the effect of LSD on spiders and their web construction.

Passion

With ASD friends, the conversation may not be as chaotic, but one particular trait that is often shared with ADHD is passion. I have found my ASD friends are more skilled at staying on topic, but often, there is still a speed and great desire to enthusiastically share our obsessions. When I was talking to autistic people for this book, I noticed how often people apologized for 'banging on'. But as I saw it, they weren't 'banging on' at all, they were just very engaged in their own particular fascinations. It became clear that this passion had often been mocked.

The rules of society seem to dictate that we should prefer the glum, the cynical and the dismissive rather than accepting and welcoming those who are highly charged with their passions. To be an enthusiast is to be frowned upon and regarded as, well, weird. Those less able to fearlessly express the joys of life, who have dulled their curiosity, will often try to smother such ebullience. Ebullience-smothering is far too common. This should concern us wherever we are on the neurodiversity spectrum. Shouldn't we all want a world where joy and progressive thoughts are not squashed by mean-spiritedness, envy and shame?

Bottling up

Some ADHD conversations are like journeys through Bosch's *Garden of Earthly Delights*. The further you travel, the greater the impossibility of pruning things back to a linear path. Your conversation will be, at best, a tesseract, a four-dimensional cube, and often just as impenetrable.

My most recent experience of such a conversation was with my writing friend Joel, who with his friend Jason created my favourite ever headline in the gorgeously rude comic *Viz*.

> *URI GELLER 'I CAN DO DOG SHITS'*
> *URI GELLER HAS STUNNED THE WORLDS OF*
> *BIOLOGY AND PARK-KEEPING BY CLAIMING*
> *HE IS ABLE TO PASS DOG STOOLS.*

THE CONVERSATION

Could a more straightforward mind ever have conjured up such a grotesque and absurd boast from the international spoon-bender?

Joel experiences conversation as if his synapses are all firing at once, lights linking up like the Vegas strip. He has learned to ignore most of them because otherwise he knows he'll knock the person he's talking to off track. He knows that, if he were to follow all the thoughts he has and express them, it would be easy for the person he is talking to to get lost and confused. Like many ADHD people, he is deeply invested in the conversation, but is connecting with anything and everything while, at the same time, trying to attend to his conversational partner because he wants to learn and understand and is hungry for new perspectives. On nights when he is among his friends, if the conversation is flagging, Joel says he's a godsend as 'that's when the "fun" version of social me' is unleashed.

When I am talking with Joel, we can both be surprised. We find our heads are fuller than we imagined and there is the discovery that things we didn't even realize were there were lurking among the synapses. 'Characteristic descriptions of the mental state in ADHD include reports of ceaseless mental activity, thoughts that are constantly on the go, or a mind constantly full of thoughts. Thoughts are experienced as uncontrolled, with multiple occurring at the same time' is how a 2016 research paper on mind wandering summarizes it.[1] I would say that is as good a description as any. It can perhaps be summed up as 'excessive spontaneous mind wandering'. The researchers looked at what they described as MEWS – the Mind Excessively Wandering Scale. I think Excessively Wandering Mind Scale might be better, but that gives you EWMS, which sounds less alluring than the cat-like MEWS.

MEWS includes the following statements and descriptors:

I find it hard to switch my thoughts off.
Because my mind is 'on the go' I have difficulty falling asleep.

> I find it difficult to think about one thing without another thought entering my mind.
> I use alcohol or other drugs to slow down my thoughts and stop constant mental chatter.
> I find my thoughts are distracting and prevent me from focusing on what I am doing.
> I try to distract myself from my thoughts by doing something else or listening to music.

Certainly, I used to be a heavy drinker. From my early twenties to my early forties, I would drink excessively on a nightly basis but I passed it off as just what you did as a working performer. Reading the statement on MEWS, it adds a level of active thought to the drinking, as if ADHD drinkers knew that the purpose of their drinking was to slow down their minds, but I would say that many do not, at least initially. I still drink every day, but far less than I used to.

The idea of distraction by music is a sweet thought, but I find music just creates more thoughts. They may be better and more useful thoughts, until you get to that song that reminds you of when Karen-Ann dumped you at the prom and you vomited in someone else's dinner jacket pocket while the covers band was playing Coldplay's 'Yellow'. I have a habit of excitedly finding a song that I love on a playlist and then fifty seconds in needing to hear another song it has reminded me of and on and on and on. That is why I would never make it as a wedding DJ, as the guests just wouldn't be able to keep up with me jumping from John Paul Young's 'Love Is in the Air' to Mudhoney's 'Touch Me I'm Sick', with John Carpenter's *Assault on Precinct 13* in between (and if you like the sound of that, book me for your wedding).

THE CONVERSATION

'I want to be part of that conversation.'

I am okay with the racing thoughts now. I think if I suddenly started experiencing a silent mind at fifty-five years old I would find it way too eerie, so I'm quite happy to sit out the noise and just wait for the inevitable never-ending silence that will come one day.

But Joel and I are the lucky ones. We have a creative outlet to let off some of the pressure. As I sift through so many odd thoughts, I can find art and jokes that I can then share with my audiences. This is not so easy for people whose lives are more restricted.

Of all the feedback I received from neurodivergent people, my favourite was probably from Beth. She told me that her friends are always saying things like, 'Why do you keep telling people that doctors used to put cocaine in their eyes before they put in contact lenses? It totally derails the conversation!' And my first thought was, *I want to be part of that conversation.*

Some like a smooth journey, but others are eager for the first derailment, the first knowledge that, whatever the original destination, it has all changed now. My advice is that we all need to throw some of the restrictive social etiquette aside and see where we might end up.

5. WORK (IS A FOUR-LETTER WORD)

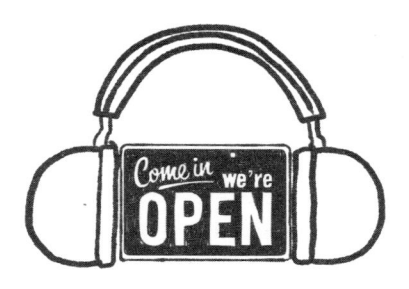

From the age of eleven, once I discovered that solitary pursuits like being washed up on a desert island weren't financially viable and could lead to gangrene, there were only two things I wanted to be – a writer or a stand-up comedian. These pursuits are not without their hierarchies, but they appeared, even then, to offer a certain freedom, and it seemed like you could spend a lot of time in your mind, which has turned out to be quite true.

Thirty-two years on, I still love the glamour of sitting alone at breakfast, in a budget hotel, dreaming up my backstory, romanticizing my travel from town to town for gigs or book events, as I peel back the seal of the individual marmalade. Over the years, I have, at times, worked in an office, but the walls soon encroached and squeezed me. I wouldn't have lasted long in that environment. I have found an escape, many others don't.

In any work world, there are a series of presumed rules, some of which are rigorously adhered to, and breaking them can put your future at risk. Like the school rules, many, when scrutinized, are only there because they are 'the done thing'. They have been passed down from one ape to another and no one quite knows why, but it is, and so it must be.

Personal space?

When I asked a group of neurodivergent people about the issues of work and its environment that make achievement more difficult, there were certain topics that came up many times. Even if you are not neurodivergent, you may well agree.

Julia opened with a rallying cry of 'Ban open plan!' For her and many others, open plan offices create an unbearable sensory overload from just too much noise and distraction. Alexandra told me that when she worked in an office, the sensory environment was unbearable. 'The noise, bright lights, general phone calls, all the screens, were awful, but the office hierarchy and politics were baffling and even worse to deal with.'

For those of us unable to tune out other people's chatter, being surrounded by five other conversations on five different topics shatters any sort of ability to focus on your own task at hand. There is also research that suggests that the desired effect of greater connection due to the shedding of walls just isn't happening. An article in the Harvard Business Review suggested, 'In a number of workplaces we have observed for research projects or consulting assignments, those structures have produced less interaction – or less *meaningful* interaction – not more.'[1]

It goes on to say that, even in the open space, an imaginary fourth wall boundary soon develops. On top of the reduction in meaningful interaction, those of us who cannot switch off our monitoring of background noise find it very hard to reach a flow state of creativity. On the rare occasions I am asked to go and work in an open plan office, I soon persuade my employers to let me work somewhere closed off, as I know I will get quadruple the work done. Also, someone like me is part of the problem in an open plan environment.

Ask anyone who has worked with me in the open plan setting of

WORK (IS A FOUR-LETTER WORD)

the BBC science unit, and they will tell you I am a terrible distractor, as all those conversations, whether on vaccines or venom or voltage, will trigger a series of paths in my brain to numerous anecdotes or questions, which I'll then voice to the room.

Julia's perfect work environment is 'a nice cosy work cubicle that shuts out distractions, and feels like your own wee den! Also, flexibility, but within clearly defined parameters/expectations, with a confident boss you can trust, who is alpha, but in an encouraging, understanding, and kind way. Is that too much to ask?' Julia's work environment is now one where the tasks are always different, constant imminent deadlines, 'enough pressure to deliver dollops of dopamine, and doesn't require hours and hours of attention focused on the same thing all the time!'

Deadlines

'WILL YOU JUST FOCUS FOR ONE GODDAM MINUTE!'

'CUT THAT DOWN TO TWENTY SECONDS AND MAYBE WE CAN MAKE A DEAL.'

A sense of jeopardy, always being on the brink of potential failure, is annoyingly vital to almost every ADHD person I know. There is no point in saying 'if you could sort it within the next month?' It needs to be 'tomorrow!' or even better 'now!'

This is why being a stand-up comedian has been perfect for me. You can't dodge the deadline. The lights come up, the audience are looking in your direction, you must start talking or miming or juggling immediately. I have spent my life saying to myself, 'Next year, I will do my tax returns four months ahead of time,' or 'Next year, I will have a fully prepared new solo show four weeks before it opens,' and never have such things happened. I now know that my limitations are where my creativity lies. The more I hem myself in with a specific script, the more I reduce my potential. I rely on having a head full of ideas and shaking them about. On the train to the show, I come up with the opening line. Then ten minutes before stage time I see something in the room that changes all that. Then, as I walk to the microphone, another notion pops into my head, and as I open my mouth, something I had not planned at all comes out. I am more passion than polish. There are plenty of people who know what they are doing, so why flood the market?

In his book *The Philosophy of Andy Warhol: from A to B and back again*, Andy Warhol wrote of how he didn't really enjoy watching professional entertainers as he knew they knew what they were doing, and he wanted something more precarious and risky. I understand this and find it suits my tastes too. For decades, my failure to 'act like a professional' was why I hated myself. Before I took to the stage, I thought I knew what I was about to do; but then, in the lights, the chaos began. Now I know that chaos is my strength. My preparation comes from living and thinking, from filling my mind. My inability to focus is fused with a dynamism that ensures I walk through the world seeing so many things – and each one causes a chain reaction of thoughts.

On a visit to Sofia in Bulgaria for a gig, I spent the first day enraptured by the doors of the city. They have some very good doors in Sofia, let me assure you. The organizers of the event had previously asked me if I could send my accompanying PowerPoint seventy-two hours in advance. I agreed, but warned them that, in the interim three days, everything would change, and so it did. At 3 p.m. on Saturday afternoon, I pressed the clicker and saw an image of the Lovell telescope. Whatever I had imagined speaking about on Thursday morning was long gone, but my brain fired up and the neural networks told a different story that was ready and appropriate about how a lasagne being microwaved in the dead of night can sometimes be confused for a signal from extraterrestrial intelligence.

Once, I would have liked to live by another set of rules, and I would fret and panic about deadlines and following other people's rules, but now, I wouldn't have it any other way.

WORK (IS A FOUR-LETTER WORD)

Energy levels and spoons

One of the most important factors when creating a workplace suitable and useful for neurodivergent people is the use of energy. This is the equation for work to energy:

$$W = K_i - K_f$$
or
$$W = \Delta K$$

W is the work done. K_i is the initial kinetic energy. K_f is the final kinetic energy. ΔK is the difference in kinetic energy. But don't worry, that's the last of that. Rather than physics, we are going to talk cutlery.

Writer Christine Miserandino came up with her influential spoon theory while eating fries and gravy in a diner with a friend. Christine has lupus, a condition that affects the immune system and can cause intense joint pain, tiredness and skin rashes. Her friend wanted to know what it felt like to be sick with lupus, not the specific physical pain, but the mental experience. Miserandino grabbed every spoon that was on or near their table and explained, 'The difference in being sick and being healthy is having to make choices or to consciously think about things when the rest of the world doesn't have to. The healthy have the luxury of a life without choices, a gift most people take for granted.' She used the spoons to explain the reduction of possibilities. She asked her friend to count the spoons. 'When you are healthy, you expect to have a never-ending supply of "spoons". But when you have to now plan your day, you need to know exactly how many "spoons" you are starting with.' She explained how you could lose a spoon – standing on the train into work, too long at the keyboard, skipping lunch, and so on. She thinks of all the spoons wasted by people in their days, and how she cannot afford to waste those spoons. She needs to end the day with one spoon left, just in case.[2]

Jamie measures out his life in spoons too. In one of our earliest conversations about neurodivergence, we discussed the problems of being neurodivergent and working for large corporations. Working as a coder, his autistic mind could achieve many things that no one else in the office could. But expressing his needs to best achieve these results, such as suggesting a small change in the office layout or lighting, he would be seen as troublesome and selfish. What his mind could give the company was rare, but with that rarity came other needs that meant the workplace required a tweak here or there. For many people, the outstanding nature of their abilities goes barely acknowledged, but anything they need to maximize the impact of those abilities becomes an outrageous demand.

Jamie sees the clocking in and clocking out culture as archaic. It might have worked when the nuts and bolts of a workplace were the actual manufacture of nuts and bolts (and rivets too), but in workplaces where the physical has made way for the virtual and the coded and a different form of solutions, the simplicity of the time sheet is no longer pragmatic. As he explains, 'There are some of us who do our best everything in these long, flowy attention tunnels. But we have a society that is increasingly designed not to create flowing attention tunnels.' The mapping of our time becomes increasingly specific. The whole concept of a nine-to-five doesn't take into account how somebody gets into the place to creatively fulfil the needs of their work.

He does not see his ADHD meds as making it easier to focus, but rather they make it easier to get into a flow state and into an attention tunnel. In an environment with too many barriers, such as noise, brightness, feelings of insecurity, or interruption, his abilities are severely hampered. Jamie now runs his own company and that has given him the opportunity to experiment with what makes him work particularly well.

WORK (IS A FOUR-LETTER WORD)

Autism can lead to burnout and fatigue. Before you come to understand your mind, you might see your burnout as failure, as opposed to a result of a period of burning brightly and possibly illuminating what others cannot. A physicist who had only been diagnosed with autism in middle age told me how she now knew how to frame the demands she needed to make when others wanted her time and expertise. She could play a major part at a conference, but it would mean she would need two days' downtime afterwards. This is not laziness, this is the necessity when you have someone with a very particular set of skills.*

The energy expended by many neurodivergent people in any interactive engagement is usually greater than average as an extra level of performance is required, along with an inability to go into an energy saving autopilot – the perpetual questioning of situations and searching for meaning and navigating the mundane rules of different environments contributes to the exhaustion. As a result, clinical psychologist Dr Megan Ann Neff breaks down the spoons idea into a neurodivergent spoon drawer: three in the executive functioning section, four in physical activity, two social spoons, two focus spoons, and so on.

As for myself, I am generally driven by taking on too much. The idea of just carrying out a single task in a day is rare. If you bought this book after an event you saw me talk at, you may well already know that, if I do a book tour, I decide I have to do three shows in three different towns every day for sixty days or more. Maybe you bought or borrowed this book after you heard about the massive cardiac arrest I suffered at gig 127 in Haverfordwest Library – thank you for the flowers. (Oh, and thanks too to that one person who brought me a hard-boiled egg and some nuts.)

Doing nothing is far more terrifying than doing everything. Jamie starts the day with ten spoons. He aims to get the most out of those

---

* Copyright Liam Neeson.

ten spoons by not dividing his day into tasks. Rather than tasks, he designs his days around tunnels. If he starts his day by getting into a flow state, then he can get lots of things done. But if he starts the day with a task hanging over him, he'll get nothing done. He uses this model to help identify the barriers and what he can effectively do about them.

> *'When I get up in the morning, I'm more focused on "how do I get into that flow state" than I am about "how do I get started on task X". So that change of lens to recognize my flowing flow states and tighten attention tunnels as the building block of my life . . . it changes everything.'*

When he does freelance work, he doesn't charge for days or hours, he charges for spoons used. The morning I speak to him, he has just completed a five-spoon project, which he describes as something really intense. Five spoons might be something involving a night in a hotel which Jamie finds tricky. Five spoons might also be three days of really fun coding, or one day of dealing with a really horrible system.

This understanding of the amount of energy he expends has no relationship to how many hours are spent working on it. Living in a world that pays people for their time assumes that every hour is the same for everyone, but that hour can be a very different reality. Jamie sees that there's an entire societal default around work and productivity, charging and freelancing. From work to shops opening and closing, to when coffee is available in the high street, the cafes that tell you that it's time to move from an Americano and a muffin to a lager and salt and vinegar crisps. Much of the pattern of our daily life is based around the assumption that hours are interchangeable and people can just turn their focus on and off.

As the great comedian Dave Allen once said:

WORK (IS A FOUR-LETTER WORD)

'You wake to the clock, you go to work to the clock, you clock-in to the clock, you clock-out to the clock, you come home to the clock, you eat to the clock, you drink to the clock, you go to bed to the clock, you get up to the clock, you go back to work to the clock . . . and when you retire, what do they give you, a fucking CLOCK!'

Jamie feels he is living a life in an environment and society that is the exact opposite of what he needs. But with the barriers identified, he has been able to consider how to overcome them and build the structures that he needs. Fortunately, he has enough power and autonomy to do that. Somebody who is eighteen years old and working in a supermarket doesn't have any chance to build that environment.

Meetings, meetings, meetings

I avoid meetings whenever possible. In my view, people who are good at meetings are often people who do nothing else. Some people are bad at meetings because they are socially anxious, uncomfortable in the blaze of bright lighting and the busyness of the room, hungry but too nervous to reach for the plate of biscuits in case they knock something over on the way or create a moment of physical social embarrassment. There are good reasons why the dyspraxic, dyslexic and autistic would rather not be penned in to someone else's minutes and pronouncements on 'the best way of us moving forward with this'.

I believe we live in a world of too many meetings – meetings about meetings to plan further meetings. We need one final meeting to work out how to end all meetings, but sadly, I fear that final meeting will be the meeting that goes on for eternity – the punishment of Satan: the devil will be in the details of the minutes.

Sadly, there are people who just love having meetings. Meetings create the illusion of having done something because you've had a meeting and that may well mean you can have another meeting to see what came out of this first meeting, and if the second meeting goes well, you can have a third meeting. In truth, many meetings don't even have biscuits any more, so there isn't even a chocolate digestive to sugar the pill.

After a corporate event, where I had briefly mentioned neurodivergence during my talk, the boss of an engineering firm approached me. He had a brilliant worker, who could achieve wonderful things, who had been diagnosed with ADHD. The problem was that this worker often missed the morning meeting.

'Does this affect his work?' I asked.

'No, but it is just that other people expect everyone to be at that meeting.'

This sounded like a case of etiquette trumping results and achievement. It sounded to me as if, for this worker at least, the meeting would actually take energy that could be used much better elsewhere. At this, you might throw your arms up in the air and say, 'Well, what if we all found an excuse to miss the meeting?' Maybe they should, maybe they shouldn't, but I don't think bringing in blanket rules for everyone when they are only useful to some people and may even be damaging for others is a solution. Blanket conformity in a world of many minds does not lead to the best results. It just saves thinking and adapting. It is convenient.

Meetings also, like overly full classrooms, often move at a slow rate that can be very frustrating for people whose minds make rapid connections. While working on a TV show, I realized three issues that needed to be dealt with to make the show more efficient and funnier. I ran them by the producer and she acknowledged that these were relevant and necessary. I was told that the TV channel that had commissioned the show were coming in for a meeting that afternoon, but as the meeting was only an hour, I would only be able to bring up one of the ideas.

'But, but, but . . .'

WORK (IS A FOUR-LETTER WORD)

I knew it would take me a total of five minutes to explain all three, rattling them off, and yet it seemed that would cause the executives' brains to melt down in horror and confusion. And this is one of the many reasons meetings are hard, because everyone is too damn slow. Too fearful of immediately grasping something, of getting excited by something, of making an immediate decision based on passion and vision.

Working from home

In a society that lacks trust and often presumes the worst, working from home has often been viewed with suspicion. The assumption is that you'll just be watching endless reruns of *Murder, She Wrote* while eating gherkins and Jelly Babies. Research often confounds this. A Chinese study of 16,000 workers over nine months found that working from home increased productivity by 13 per cent.[3] Unfortunately, the Scrooge-ish nature of our overlords and their inability to believe we will be able to resist Angela Lansbury means progress towards working from home has been slow, and many companies have been zealous in persuading employees to return to their offices after the COVID lockdown.

Opinions from both ADHD and autistic workers I spoke to included:

> 'Working from home is great for me, there's much less noise and distraction. But if I had to go back (and I will one day) my noise-cancelling headphones with focus music will be invaluable again.'
>
> 'I kinda miss the company but schlepping to work (and the getting dressed as a disabled person) is hard work in itself!'

For Sooz, working from home made it possible for her to get back to earning a living again. She no longer had to cope with long, draining commutes, or 'the oppressive office environment of distraction, meetings that could be emails and pointless office politics'. Working from home means she is in control of her environment and her working hours too. If she is having a good day, she can do an extra hour, then when having a bad day, she can step away and just let it take its toll. 'The flexibility takes the worry away.' She doesn't believe she could go back to an office now. Before the pandemic, she hadn't worked since 2016 and thought she'd never work again. The future looked bleak. Since working from home has become more normal and employers have become more flexible, things have fallen into place.

Whether neurodivergent or neurotypical, the continued notion that you must GO to work seems weird to me. This is all very well if you are a steelworker, as furnaces and smelters are often hard to construct in spare bedrooms or back gardens, but so much communication can be done without all travelling to the same building and so much time can be saved. The ability to control the environment that you are working in brings many improvements to so many people's lives.

Email

Of course working from home means that you have to stay in touch with the rest of your work colleagues and share your ideas with them through means other than shouting across the open plan office.

I have found it is important for me to try to catch a thought and keep it, however I can. It is no good me saying, 'I'll remember to do that when I get home,' because it will soon be lost on the turbulent sea of all the other thoughts I wasn't expecting on my journey. I will remember, with a start, at 2 a.m. and immediately commit to doing it the first moment I wake up. This carousel will continue for some time, with a possibility that it will go on for eternity.

Perhaps the fastest way, if you have the technology, is to record a voice memo on your phone. You can also text yourself. Halfway through the last sentence, I went to do that with my phone, but there was another text about a poetry event that had come in which needed me to find an email, but there was a new email from someone else about a silent movie event involving a cat and a canary and that reminded me that I hadn't given the friend who I created a musical with about giant crabs a quote for his autobiography and . . . Where am I?

What I am aware of now is that when I see an email, I must reply *immediately* or accept there is a high percentage chance it will not be answered at all. When I give my email address to people who want me for something, I will always say, 'If I haven't replied within five minutes of you sending this, send it again in a few days and do not think I am deliberately ignoring you. Resend until I reply.' I know that sounds bothersome, but I need people to know that I am genuinely interested in their library or charity event or science fiction poetry and not blanking them on purpose. Also, I give my email to almost everyone, as every project they mention or charity they represent sounds interesting and exciting and I am usually in a manic, post-gig state. I also ask people to put the vital information of any email in the first sentence as each further word creates further chance of disconnection and distraction.

Autonomy

I know I am privileged to have the autonomy I have, much of it coming from a secure background, being white, and middle class, and male. Also, the career I have pursued is one that allows me greater autonomy than most. I have just enough success to be choosey. I don't have to do every job that comes my way. I am able to take jobs that pay less or do not pay at all, so long as there are enough jobs that I can take every now and again to top things up. I think hanging around with neurodivergent people has helped me battle against my lust for capitalist fulfilment and see through the necessary delusions to maintain the correct level of anxiety.

If I become richer, then I might end up at that point where my wealth becomes my defining feature and I will have to make more and more so I can indulge in rare pâté from exploded wildfowl liver, hair weaves made from the locks of children reared on mink farms, and a big helicopter.

On a train journey once with Joanne Harris, the author of *Chocolat*, we talked of the strangeness of those wealthy artists who have a fixed rate. You either pay their fee or you can't afford them, but then, as an artist, what experiences might you be turning down? Money brings with it its own restrictions. But when there are people making money from you, you should be paid properly, and that doesn't happen for enough people. We have to work out a careful balance between fair remuneration and greed. In many of the places I have worked, I have seen the imbalance.

So what are you worth?

It is a great trick of contemporary capitalism to give vast remuneration to those at the top, while allowing those same people to tell those below them that it is rude to ask for too much. While we have all perhaps been made to feel that way, if you are already plagued with low self-worth, that will affect how much you believe you are worth monetarily in the working world. Many people, through the anxiety they carry and feelings of low self-esteem, are either manipulated by the system or just far too ready to accept far less than they should be receiving, or both. Many of us are ashamed to bring up the subject of money with our employers for fear of being perceived as arrogant enough to think we are worth something more.

For a neurodivergent mind, having such conversations can bring even more anxiety from the fear that we will misread the situation and get things wrong. Even though I have become far more comfortable and confident with who I am over the past few years and am getting better at this, the embarrassment of discussing remuneration remains. I have performed in the past for free when others have received thousands, just because I have been paralysed about bringing up the subject of money. The mixture of a desire to make people happy and a sense that I don't really deserve the money produces embarrassment and silence. If you think you are shit, then you accept people undermining you and undervaluing you.

You can also reframe yourself as an impediment, a weight around the company's neck. After all, look at the fuss that was made when you politely asked to work different hours, or left the office party early. You are the factor that stops something being better. Your performance is always at fault. Many neurodivergent people are adept at analysing the minutiae of every task they do. However well it may appear that they have completed their job, they will find the fault and magnify it until it becomes a crater, always presuming someone else would have done it far better.

The confidence illusion

During a recent radio recording, I had a first-time guest on the show talking about an important scientific debate about asteroids, but we ended up talking about whether dogs were better than cats. Dogs won, whatever the cat people say. After the show, I sensed that the guest felt disappointed with her contribution, that she didn't feel she had been good enough. I said nothing that night, but a few days later I sent her a message saying she had been excellent and that I was worried she may have been worried. She admitted she had been, and we talked about what our self-critical voices tell us and the reality of such situations. Making such conversations open, allowing them to not be off-limits, allows for a real sense of freedom and release.

Similarly, on a major tour of North America, I could tell that the tour manager was having trouble dealing with a star who was not obedient when it came to doing what the producer wanted. I sensed her anxiety. I explained to her that I often experienced anxiety and that I understood how difficult this must have been for her, and we tried to work out a system that would lighten the pressure and stave off the black dog of stress and depression. Self-knowledge gained through understanding our neurodivergence can also give us the tools to see more clearly what others may be fighting with.

Lisa Blower, author of *It's Gone Dark over Bill's Mother's*, was stage managing the literature stage at Latitude Festival. I had been putting on events all weekend, and towards the end of Sunday, she said to me, 'I wish I had your confidence. It is amazing how you just interact with so many people.' It was a lovely thing to say, though it did not reflect my own internal experience. Throughout every supposedly confident interaction, my internal heckler was telling me that the people I was talking to thought I was rubbish. They were appalled that I was talking to them, and it was barely believable that I had been employed to be there when there were so many better people available. It was entirely conceivable to me that every one of them left our conversations and, as soon as they presumed they were out of earshot, said, 'That man is so awful.'

The energy of my confidence was powered by my perpetual anxiety. Despite the success of the radio show *The Infinite Monkey Cage*, I used to be hollered at by my internal heckler throughout every show. 'You shouldn't have said that joke there. That idea didn't go down well enough. People only want to hear Brian Cox. You're ruining the show. Everyone knows you are clueless about string theory. That scientist has never met anyone as stupid as you are. The show was brilliant until you opened your mouth,' and on and on and on.

Yet while all that ruckus was going on inside my head, the healthier part of my mind was making up jokes and ideas and segues. I was totally immersed in creating the show, while at the

WORK (IS A FOUR-LETTER WORD)

same time, I was also totally immersed in dealing with someone throwing bottles – a superposition of creativity and self-hate. The plethora of connections was both the problem and the solution. It was like living in the online comments section of a newspaper.

With an ADHD mind, the rapid-fire emotional circuitry lacks any delicacy in its dealings with your feelings, and so a minor work error can plunge you straight into desperation. And as we know, the negative is always right, and the positive thoughts are an arrogant indulgence.

Once I started to understand how an ADHD mind might work, I began to accept that I could not lobotomize my own mind into a form where the sluice gates of my neural pathways would flow evenly and predictably. I could not train my mind to be 'normal', but I could reframe my battle with it. I could see what it positively gave me, and I could find the advantages rather than seek a cure. I could start to feel satisfied with what my mind brought to the work environment, things other ways of thinking would not be able to achieve. I was able to stop inflating my faults to the point of suffocation and use this new breathing space to create positively.

Before that, not only did I often feel I was not the best person for the job, someone who had been far luckier than they deserved, but I would often work hard to persuade people not to employ me in the first place. I was going to work with one of the comedy heroes of my youth, Eric Idle, on a TV musical. I was so certain that he must have put me in the show under some sort of duress or obligation that on the first day of rehearsals I approached him and explained that I had worked out how my part could be removed without damaging the narrative and exactly what needed to be done so the plot could flow without me. This now seems both rude and silly on my part.

I am now arrogant enough to believe I am actually pretty good at some things. I am aware of my limitations, but I am also prepared to acknowledge that, on occasion, I really might be the right person for the job, and if I am not, then I am going to take it anyway and have fun despite their poor judgement in employing me.

To conceal or not to conceal

And yet it can be difficult to be honest about your neurodivergence at work as this can hand over a weapon, a reason to be dismissed and a reason to be patronized.

William wasn't diagnosed with ADHD until his sixties, and he believes that diagnosis would have excluded him from virtually every job he has ever had. He told me that he thought his employers knew he was a bit odd, but neither they nor him could put a finger on why that was. He got the right results, so he remained, but he focused hard on masking. He feels that diagnosis without accommodation in the past would have been quite counterproductive, but he believes that people do 'get it' more now. And most importantly, he can now make sense of 'a hitherto insoluble puzzle'.

Before his diagnosis, Matt found he was in a battle against the idea that you are meant to specialize. Neurodivergence can often mean you need regular hits of change while society says that it really is best to follow one path in your work life. Otherwise, in job interviews, you'll find prospective employers asking, 'So why do you want to work in the ice-cream flavour development department when your previous jobs have been a market gardener specializing in watercress, a road manager for a death-metal band, a motorway service station designer and a Roy Orbison impersonator?'

Matt says:

> 'Jack of all trades isn't bad, but for years I thought I was a failure because I switched careers four times (with a fifth in progress aged forty-seven). Luckily, the programming wasn't strong enough to stop me from actually doing it, but how that odd-seeming CV

WORK (IS A FOUR-LETTER WORD)

interacts with the general neurodiverse feeling of failure isn't very pretty sometimes. I've been successful by any count in most of my career choices, but unless I sternly deal with my self-talk, I can feel otherwise. As I've got older, I've been very grateful that I followed my nose to what felt interesting to me rather than trying to force myself into the neurotypical steady path.'

Failure falls on fertile ground when it lands on the neurodivergent. Few of us revel in our own failure, but some, in the bloom of success, will rip through the rose beds until they find the smallest weed of failure, and soon it will cover them like ivy, but twice as itchy.* Many, across the spectrum of neurodiversity, are wearing dung-tinted spectacles and this can make the workplace very challenging.

This is something many people feel with different levels of intensity. Impostor syndrome, as it is known, is the recurring thought that you are the only one who has not got a clue what you are doing. Concealing what you believe to be your incompetence can be exhausting in itself. It can also make it easier for you to be manipulated, work longer hours, and get less pay. By not feeling you're good enough, you will always find it hard to ask for what is actually due to you, never mind asking for a wage increase. Many companies operate in a subtly abusive way. They want you to believe that you are lucky to be working for them rather than they are lucky to have you.

Neurodivergent people can often be the easiest to manipulate. They already have battles navigating the world, following social cues, obeying rules, and listening to a voice that underlines their inability to be a proper human.

---

* I continue to torture metaphors, but I am looking at roses as I write this.

NORMALLY WEIRD AND WEIRDLY NORMAL

Other people's stories

Becky's answer to the question of the pitfalls and positives of working as a neurodivergent was simply 'perfectionism and perfectionism'.

I have spoken to many autistic people who often struggle with the impossibility of ever completing a task because it fails to meet the perfection they imagine can exist, like Plato seeking perfect solids. Poet and author Tim Clare told me:

> 'I guess the pitfalls are more salient to me: perfectionism, which can paralyse me so I can't do anything at all, and making stuff that might not connect with people because it's not relatable, because my way of thinking is unusual. But of course both these things can also be strengths – high standards and originality.'

Katie, an artist and comedian, never wants to finish a project whether an artwork, book, poem or play because then it will be finished. 'I don't think my writing or creative skills can do my ideas justice, and as long as they remain incomplete, they still have boundless potential and scope. Sounds really weird, I know.' This seems common for many people, however their brain may pivot. We are relentless tweakers, though some of us spend more time than others delaying the moment of confrontation with the inevitable deadline and some people spend far more time obsessing on how much better it could have been.

Beth, an artist and puppet builder, needs to finish things there and then or they add to her large pile of 'will finish someday' projects. Because of that she works fast. 'But I'm always surrounded by self-perceived failure. I've occasionally had hyperfixations (building laser cut things and some specific crafting things) which have bucked this trend, but they do get all-consuming.' She gets 'really drained' by being bored or annoyed, which was a particular problem when she worked in admin. Boredom and monotony are vile devils to ADHD people. The mind is always seeking novelty.

Esme told me, 'If I just do things my way, it's often incomprehensible without significant explanation to others.' She must adapt to the 'norm' or else she creates ten times the workload. I have the good fortune that I ended up in a career where being inscrutable can be presumed to be artistic intention. This may be another reason why I find work easier than day to day living and why I do so much of it, as a way to put off failing at the normal tasks.

Bob is similar. He is a writer and finds that his brain very easily makes connections between completely unrelated things, which is really handy for writing magazine features that go in sometimes delightfully unexpected directions, but he finds it less convenient when he has to buy the same sandwich from the same shop at the same time every day for a week to stave off a nuclear war. This creating of an unrelated catastrophe due to an unrelated action is very much akin to the behaviour of avoiding stepping on the cracks in the pavement. This thinking may be why obsessive compulsive disorder is sometimes diagnosed as ADHD and vice versa. In a 2014 paper, 'The neurobiological link between OCD and ADHD', it was estimated that between 8 and 25 per cent of people diagnosed with OCD are also ADHD.[4] It is the most common co-occurring condition with ADHD. Dr Neff, who was late-diagnosed ADHD and autistic, compares the two. Seeing the ADHD issue as 'time blindness', which yet again, comes from the difficulty with regulating attention and focus, and with executive function. While for OCD, 'obsessions and compulsions can make attention, focus, and following through on tasks difficult. A person may also struggle with timeliness and time management if they spend copious amounts of time engaging in compulsions'.

For Robin (not me, I haven't started talking about myself in the third person quite yet), the issue is not creativity but the paperwork that it might entail. It is the speed in which a neurodivergent mind can say, 'Sorry, but I am not aligned to deal with instruction manuals or documents for registering things and that includes registering my show for a festival.' Robin sees the downs and ups of his ADHD mind. Yes, they can have huge problems filling in the forms to register their show *CatGPT* because they 'genuinely cannot fathom their wretched online form'. But on the plus side, 'Nobody else would've come up with a head-bending interactive show involving an actual dead cat with a modular synthesizer, Dreamies, projection, an AI brain and a minibar. What can possibly go wrong?!'

Filling in forms, whether autistic, ADHD or dyslexic, is frequently a nightmare. This is not to say that there are lots of people who get a kick out of the frequently Kafkaesque qualities of document design. Simplicity is an anathema to whoever it is who lives in the secret bunker where form designers cackle away at our agony. Advice on better design for forms for autistic people includes using muted colours NOT vibrant contrasting colours. Writing in plain language. Using simple sentences and bullet points, not walls of language, and creating simple and consistent layouts. In 'The Buckland Review of Autism and Employment', ambiguous interview questions and application forms were found to be keeping autistic people out of work.[5] Many employers have been resistant to finding alternative ways of recruiting staff. Dr James Cusack, chief executive of research charity Autistica, said:

> 'To be their best and to ensure they can get the best out of their whole workforce, including autistic people, employers need to change the way that they recruit and support staff . . . This is not about reasonable adjustments for a small number of people – it's about changes that benefit everyone, because we all think and work differently.'[6]

WORK (IS A FOUR-LETTER WORD)

Other suggestions to improve job applications are having tick-boxes in applications instead of free-form text-boxes and being able to receive interview questions in advance.

Neil, like many people with ADHD, does not need all the instructions however much an employer or work colleague may want to give them. He sees the benefits of his jigsaw puzzle mind. His mind jumps from point a to z and the in-between of the puzzle snaps together. When a trainer tells him he hasn't given him all the details yet, Neil will meticulously explain the entire project to them without having been given up to 50 per cent of the instructions and nail it every time. He says that people are dumbfounded by this. The negatives kick in for him the moment the stress does. When a stress overload occurs – and it can be from the slightest failure of understanding or communication – even the ability to spell a simple word is vaporized. Similarly, I can be in a flow state moving at incredible speed, but when an impediment occurs, the implosion can be all-encompassing.

Alice, who works in academia, believes she is on the autistic spectrum and finds the benefits are that she can focus really intensely on something, especially writing, and get something really polished very quickly. And because she's never mastered academese, she can make it really clear at lots of levels too (just what we want – clear language).

On the downside, if she doesn't fall into intense focus quickly, she can procrastinate and panic for days, 'or years, depending on the situation'. She can totally misread the room and waste a lot of effort writing something that wasn't what was being looked for. Similarly, she can find it impossible to adapt to the style people want, such as if they want something very dry and aimed at grant funders rather than a curious member of the public. She believes she can really fail to respect or devote enough energy to a task if she doesn't think there's any point in doing it.

NORMALLY WEIRD AND WEIRDLY NORMAL

A creative mind

Dyslexic scientific experiment designer Fran Scott nearly killed me once. Walking in the dark, backstage at the Hammersmith Apollo while hosting an event, I fell over a wide selection of large, long metal pipes and clattered about just as an astronaut on stage was trying to talk about exiting the Earth's atmosphere.

Fran worked for the Royal Institution for many years, building experiments for their Christmas Lectures among other adventures, and the pipes belonged to Fran and were part of her show. She describes the benefit of her neurodivergent brain as the creativity which perpetually buzzes around it and how it gives her the ability to solve problems swiftly. She has to truly understand something to remember it. Which means she properly understands a fair bit. Because she has always had to work harder to ensure comprehension, she believes this is why she is not afraid of hard work. She sees the pitfalls of her brain as its inbox gets full too easily 'because everything comes with so many appendices', and sometimes, she just has to fall asleep to get everything filed away properly.

It is my lack of focus that has given me a career; it is my lack of focus that has nearly destroyed my career and at times made it hard to keep on going. Wise people such as Professor Brian Cox sometimes class what comes from my mouth as 'gibberish', but it is not nonsense, it is just too much for some. Cox, who can grasp the inscrutable quantum behaviour of subatomic particles and understand any event horizon crossing, finds me quite incomprehensible.

But a mind such as mine makes it easy to perform to a live audience, but harder to write books. When I began writing this one, I wanted it to reflect what my mind was doing as I wrote. I wanted to include all the diversions I indulged in, such as the periods of time where I stopped writing mid-sentence to watch online footage of

WORK (IS A FOUR-LETTER WORD)

classic tap-dancing routines by Gregory Hine and Sammy Davis Jr, or the sudden fascination I would develop with books called *What Would Jesus Eat?*, or pondering which was my favourite rendition of 'Stormy Weather', or considering entrances and exits for fictional characters I had suddenly conjured up, or just how wide a wormhole could be, or my designs for a malicious lemonade machine, or deeply considering the thought processes I imagine a death watch beetle might have and how I might explain to others how I came to such conclusions. It was beyond dizzying. One day, I will write that book, or it will write me.

Suffice to say, when the editor saw what I was trying to do, there was a hastily assembled meeting and my chance to accidentally create something more confusing than *Finnegans Wake* was rapidly curtailed. You have to have written at least one bona fide 1,040-page classic of English literature before you are allowed to do that sort of thing.

The relentlessness of ideas that ADHD people experience means that, in truth, the words 'attention deficit' are unhelpful. There is no shortage of attention – it is just working in a different time frame to many of the people around you. That attention is attempting to attend to everything that is pinging around the brain. Ellie Middleton, who was diagnosed with ADHD and autism when she was twenty-four, describes ADHD as 'not about a deficit of attention, but instead being a dysregulated attention system'.

Since discovering my own mind is ADHD, I haven't wasted nearly as much time in berating myself and have instead spent far more time working out how to make the best of myself. I decided that at fifty-two years old my executive functions may be stuck in their ways, but that didn't mean that I needed to be.

Where was I?

It seems to me that far too many neurodivergent people are being forced to work in environments designed for a so-called 'average' person who barely exists, and that far too many negative judgements are made when this is questioned. Whether neurodivergent or neurotypical, we all gain by listening to the needs and desires of employees and creating environments which mean that work is not a daily dread.

I find it so exciting to be surrounded by people who are perpetually generating connections, seeing things that others missed, creating things they weren't expecting. It builds new worlds and recolours the old worlds. We must embrace the notion that the expected is not always the best. It is important for neurodivergent people to realize that their ability to confound and surprise is often not their failure, but the wonder of a mind that fizzes so much and with such passion that it is actually delivering more to the world.

6. HOARDING, COLLECTING AND OBSESSIONS

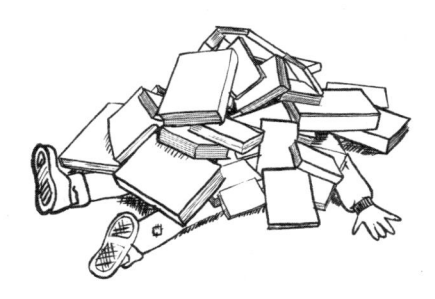

Should you ever read in some quiet corner of the internet that I died accidentally after a vast pile of books fell on me, don't believe a word of it. It was murder. The most likely reason that one day I will be divorced and die alone is my passion for collecting, collecting, collecting. My bedroom is filled with books and memorabilia I have collected over the years, and it spills out further across our not very big house.

I am not being flippant when I write that many of the greatest tensions in the relationship I have with my wife come from my excitement about strange books and archaic magazines I discover filled with technicolour illustrations of 1950s pavlovas that I insist must become mine. I try to stop. I wish I could get rid of them all, but I just can't seem to and so our house can be a very cold place.

By the way, the reason I refer to 'my bedroom' above is that I sleep in my own room in the attic because:

A. I snore like the last buffalo;
B. I have huge and unruly stacks and stacks of printed and scribbled-on material which I frequently turn to in the night;
C. Despite every evening being sure I will be under a duvet by

NORMALLY WEIRD AND WEIRDLY NORMAL

11 p.m., I seem to find it impossible to go to bed before 2 a.m.*

The physical impacts of a neurodivergent mind can often raise problems for flatmates and partners alike. And it is not always an easy division between the notion that ADHD means chaos and ASD means incredibly tidy.

Mountains of mess

I'm not a hoarder, honest. I just need stuff *everywhere* and will find more stuff to acquire in every town I visit. My hoarding begins with an excited and elevated feeling that I have to have something, which may well be what is termed 'hypomania'. It's a word that was totally alien to me until comic book artist Jamie McKelvie saw a photo of my bedroom and said, 'You know what that is? Hypomania.' It is an 'apparently non-contextual elevation of mood that contributes to a persistently disinhibited behaviour' and it is the state I am often in when I am in a junk shop or bookshop. I find one fascinating thing and, somehow, that one fascinating thing then enchants so many other objects in the store, and I'm beyond excitement and all judgement is gone. Ask me why I have dragged them home and I may have no answer, but in that moment of enchantment they all had to be mine. I become intensely obsessed.

With piles of stuff comes mountains of mess. When it comes to neatness, tidiness is Tokyo and I am Godzilla. I must destroy order. It is not that I want to, but it is uncontrollable – it is the beast in me.

My friend Stuart is very ordered. His CD collection is carefully boxed around themes – albums recorded by musicians who named their children after players in the 1930s jazz scene, singers who walked into deserts and did not return for over three months, bands that use conches, and some just rather dully based on the geographical

---

* Another impact of having an overactive mind.

HOARDING, COLLECTING AND OBSESSIONS

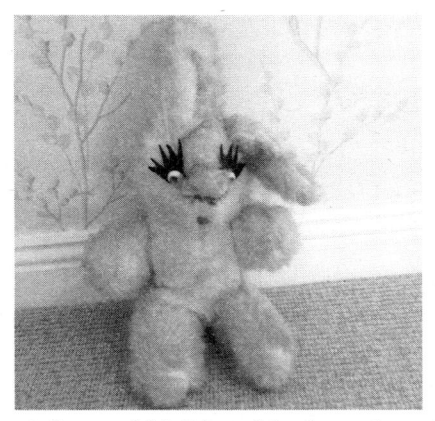

A profoundly weird toy rabbit I found in the attic and had to share.

locations of record labels. This is why, when people say, 'I think I am a bit autistic, my record collection is in alphabetical order,' we can be suspicious. That is merely pragmatism, not autism.

I used to think order like Stuart's would be possible for me. I've tried it. But then I would be halfway through ordering all my music, either based on month of release or longitude of the pressing plant or whether the bassist lived in a property once owned by a necromancer, and I would reach a record that would seem impossible to place in the categories I had created, and with that, all order would be washed away like a sandcastle in the face of the encroaching tide. This is the reason I have spent much of my life galloping around my house shouting out for objects that I cannot find, calling lost books and tax documents to me as if they were sheepdogs.

Twice a year I have a tidy desk, sometimes for up to forty-eight hours, but then things begin to gravitate and stack up. Every time I have tidied my desk, I really, really, *really* believe that it will stay that way, but as I look away, the entropy fairy comes and fires a leaf blower at it. Similarly, my glasses are always dirty, though I have no idea why. I will wipe them with the finest alcohol-infused cloth until they glisten, then within five minutes, I find that a syrup-fingered goblin has smeared their way across them.

NORMALLY WEIRD AND WEIRDLY NORMAL

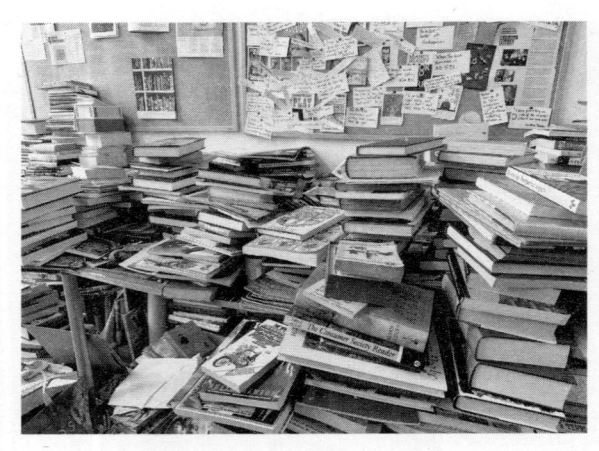

My typically tidy office. Entropy increased shortly afterwards.

I know a lot of disordered people, so I thought we were normal. I think we *are*. For me it is the ordered who are weird. Their habitat lacks the element of surprise – the 1953 leaflet about Avebury's stone circles and henge that I brought home from a jumble sale or that dead mouse you didn't know had died squashed under an encyclopedia of prog rock that toppled off a shelf.

When I was thinking of moving house, I had the opportunity to see inside other people's homes and smell all the bread they had been baking.* It surprised me how little stuff so many people had. Sure, I know you hide your stuff when you are trying to sell your house, especially the meathooks and bone saws, but these houses were so bereft of 'things' and 'stuff' – so few books, so few records, so few vast stacks of music magazines from the 1980s, so few music boxes that played the Harry Lime theme from *The Third Man*, so few wooden monkey heads that were former tobacco holders.

The houses I saw had so few shelves. The shelves they did have were underused, just small bits of glassware with maybe a photograph

---

* Estate agent tip 101: do not make a house smell like a butcher's. That's just creepy.

of their daughter's graduation or the husband beaming in a wetsuit in Barbados, sometimes holding a dogfish. That was that. Barely worth a shelf at all. Oh, the weight I could burden those shelves with . . . They could feel truly useful for the first time.

It is all very well following the nineteenth-century artist's advice of 'have nothing in your home apart from that which is useful and that which is beautiful', but what if you find beauty in almost everything . . . and everything could have a use? I can imagine there will eventually be a use for that box of antique prosthetic hands I bought in a junk shop that looked interesting. My alibi is always that I will make a story or something creative for my shows from the nonsense I empty out of my rucksack after a day at the flea market. Every object seems to contain stories, and I need and love stories.

Doom bags

Have you heard of the Doom bag? Steve, another ADHDer, introduced me to this idea. He told me that social media is full of ADHD people opening and discussing their Doom bags.

These are the bags that 'you stuff shit in and shove in the shed during the frantic tidy up before you have visitors so that they assume you haven't just tidied up'. Steve has Doom bags going back to when T'Pau were number one in the charts. They remind me of the time my wife said to me, 'You are the kind of person who will be found dead surrounded by bags of stuff.' A typical tote bag in my room, and there are many, may contain some leaflets given to me on a march about restoring nature, a book of Yoko Ono's art instructions, a facsimile of Vincent Price's cookbook, *Cooking Price-Wise*, a theatre programme for a 1997 production of *Krapp's Last Tape*, a selection of pencils, a notebook with half a poem in it, and some oatcakes and a complimentary energy bar handed to me at a train station. At least, that was what was in the nearest one to me as I was writing this.

NORMALLY WEIRD AND WEIRDLY NORMAL

Many have Doom boxes too. Doom does not mean doom. Doom actually stands for 'Didn't Organize Only Moved'. It's a solution for all those times you've been asked, 'Are you really sure you want to keep that thing and not just take it down to the rubbish tip?' And you have fought tooth and nail to keep it. You might not look at it or need it for months, but until you do, you know where it is.

Though the Doom box definition is meant to be for the box that just follows you from house to house, I think many people have Doom boxes even if they are not peripatetic. To me, it is a box of things your imagination could not quite find a reason to keep, but your emotions could not find a reason to part with. I have found many such boxes in my dad's house since he died in 2023. With his death, they have become puzzle boxes: 'What even is that?'

A friend of mine told me about her dad leaving one of his Doom boxes behind when he moved house. Some days after the new owners had moved in, he remembered he'd left it behind. It was a box containing a large jar of sulphuric acid and a carrier bag of asbestos. He rang to tell the new owners.

'Yes, we have found that!' they replied with angry frustration. It was a short phone call.

Obsessions and manias

Similarly, as well as hoarding things, I can have brief but intense fascinations that must be sated. I become overwhelmed by a sudden impulsivity and obsession.

I might see a documentary or an interview with someone and immediately say to myself, 'I have to know everything about that person and read everything they have ever written.' I have an entire shelf of books by the Slovenian philosopher Slavoj Žižek because I once saw a film of him walking around a rubbish tip in a high-vis jacket commenting on Western consumer society and mocking the pornography he found among the rubbish sacks.[1] As

HOARDING, COLLECTING AND OBSESSIONS

he disparagingly lifted up a damp and torn magazine from the dump he declared, 'You call this pornography?' and my fate was sealed. I had to have everything he had written, even the books he had written about Hegel for which I had none of the intellectual tools to understand. Almost all of those books are unread. But they are there, waiting, and still full of possibility and my good intentions to read them.

I once read a small piece about Søren Kierkegaard and thought, I must read his masterwork *Either/Or* right now. That was in 1992. I think I am at page seven. Not all obsessions vanish just as the books arrive. A few bloom, and it is those few blooms that justify my lack of reason.

New manias are constantly replacing old ones. Each time, I am sure that this time I will read the book all the way through and listen to all the records and watch all the films I have just ordered. Twenty-four-hour online shopping makes this situation even worse because everything is immediately accessible and order-able. This compulsive behaviour is frequently observed in those with bipolar disorder and ADHD. A two-part study by the Academy of Research and Improvement for the Solent NHS Trust (now Hampshire and Isle of Wight Healthcare NHS Trust) has found links between bipolar disorder and compulsive spending. It highlighted that 'compulsive spending . . . was increased over time by higher dependency and achievement cognitions, lower mindfulness and lower self-esteem'.[2] The report also noted that this can create a vicious cycle, because the compulsive spending leads to anxiety due to overspending and possibly going into debt caused by the manic phase of purchasing.

Dr Thomas Richardson, one of the report's authors, who is bipolar himself, said:

'When I was manic aged eighteen, I went into a shop and bought five African djembe drums at once. To my friends and family, this seemed like a random purchase, like I had just seen them

and liked the look of them, but actually, in my mind, it linked to a very unrealistic and impulsive business plan I had to set up a recording studio. I was trying to make myself some money for starting university, but I ended up getting into debt.[3]

Leah Milner, a money and mental health journalist with bipolar disorder, has also written of how the manic purchases that seem random can come with the illusion of a plan. She wanted to write an article about how you could buy a whole new work wardrobe from charity shops, so this justified her spending a lot of money on second-hand clothes. Her thinking was disordered, so many of the shoes she bought were not even the right size. She loves painting and thought some of the random purchases she made 'such as a top hat or crockery' could be props that she could use for still life scenes. 'In that context the purchases do not seem so strange, but it was the compulsion to buy so many things with only the slightest hint of an idea and the scale of the spending that was problematic,' she wrote and a bell as big as Notre Dame rang in my head.

So many things seem so full of potential. I compulsively need to purchase things believing that this weight of objects will help the birth process of ideas. I have sometimes even knowingly bought a book I own already, believing that having a second copy will somehow make it more likely that I will read it.

According to a 2022 survey undertaken by YouGov, people with ADHD are four times more likely to frequently overspend, and for 60 per cent of them, this has a direct impact on their ability to manage money day to day.[4] All of this is great news for capitalism, but terrible news for neurodivergent individuals trying to balance their bills.

I am fortunate that the relentless lessons in parsimony taught to me by my father mean that I have a deep anxiety about money, made more pertinent by being self-employed for my whole adult life. That said, my father's care with money seemed to decline with age. In every cupboard in his house, behind his Doom boxes, we

HOARDING, COLLECTING AND OBSESSIONS

found another stack of random objects that we had no idea he had purchased, often still in their packaging. Most of this was from the last ten years of his life when he was at first housebound looking after our mother, and then housebound due to his own fragility.

In those years, he had built up quite a collection of commemorative coins. Not the ones that are absolute tat and are advertised on daytime television by retired news anchors: 'this gold-effect 27-gramme doubloon commemorates the forty-third anniversary of the Cold War/the launch of the *Marie Celeste*/the release of *The Revenge of the Pink Panther*'. He had good taste until the end. All the coins had remained in their boxes, and though my eldest sister and I usually brought in his mail, we had never noticed the boxes finding their way into his house. Canny until the end too.

He was always staving off boredom, always curious. In the last few months of his life, I was pretty sure he was departing because he thought the boredom had started to win. Boredom is my archnemesis too, and so far, he usually loses (yes, in my mind, boredom is a HE). Men can class their hoarding as collecting. It becomes a hobby, not a possible disorder. 'I just happen to be a keen collector of stamps; newspapers; yoghurt pots; sliced ham packaging; heads that have dropped off cheap, poor-quality, mid-Victorian taxidermy; birds' eggs; hot water bottles; and used razors.'

At my dad's funeral, I based his eulogy around some of the objects we had found as we had started sorting out the house. The stuffed stoat, the wren whose wing had accidentally been vacuum-cleaned off when it had become dusty, old exercise books with advice he had written as a teenager on how to ascend cliffs in the hope of photographing puffins, and a signed copy of *Penthouse* magazine from 1969. I found that the pulpit shelf was not wide enough to hold such a menagerie of objects, and I had to lean against the stoat quite heavily to prevent an avalanche for much of the eulogy. I can particularly recommend using vintage erotica in your eulogy if you can find any in your dead relative's collection, as it is a superb icebreaker at the wake.

NORMALLY WEIRD AND WEIRDLY NORMAL

Hoarding is not specifically male, though it is often considered to be. One of the best pieces of work about that narrow divide between collecting and hoarding is Carol Morley's *Typist Artist Pirate King*, a partly fictionalized look at the life of Audrey Amiss, an outsider artist diagnosed as bipolar schizophrenic. Amiss's archive is really the collection of a life. It totals eighty heavy boxes and includes 50,000 sketches, her paintings and diaries. She wrote thousands of letters to people ranging from the Queen to Mother Teresa to McDonald's customer services. She also made scrapbooks with the packaging from all the food and drink she consumed and noted her thoughts about the designs on the wrappers. Morley writes about Amiss, 'She wrote that a bowl of Kellogg's Frosties "resembles a storm in a tea cup", that the illustration on a Quavers packet "suggests a haircut".'[5]

The rise of inaccessibility

The NHS defines hoarding as 'where someone acquires an excessive number of items and stores them in a chaotic manner, usually resulting in unmanageable amounts of clutter. The items can be of little or no monetary value'. Fortunately, that can't be me, as my vast pile of *Man, Myth and Magic* magazines from the early seventies are still worth their original cover price at the very least, and some may be worth even more than six pence.*

I am pretty certain that I am a chaotic collector. My tastes are wide but still too specific . . . or are they? What would my house look like if I lived alone?

The crossing point from having 'too much stuff' to hoarding is deemed to be having so much stuff that rooms, including possibly the bathroom or kitchen, become too full to be accessible (not there yet) and where 'the clutter is causing significant distress or

---

* Let's be honest, we all know I am looking at £4 plus *each*.

HOARDING, COLLECTING AND OBSESSIONS

negatively affecting the quality of life of the person or their family – for example, they become upset if someone tries to clear the clutter and their relationship suffers'.[6] I probably am pretty much teetering on that line now and sometimes falling over onto the other side of it.

I do battle to reduce the piles from time to time, especially when I can see it is causing anxiety and distress. The irony is that collecting things obsessively can be caused by anxiety and distress, and takes hold because it creates a certain form of order in a wild world of uncertainty, which is a common feeling in neurodivergence. But just as the collecting brings order, should you share your space with anyone else, you may be pushing them into the very condition you are trying to escape from.

Often thousands of books will leave the house in a year, though how many thousand new ones come in is debatable. So far today, I have purchased all twelve issues of *Art in Focus* from 1974 (bound); a biography of Chris Sievey, the creator of Frank Sidebottom, the helium-voiced pop legend with a papier mâché head; another book on the holographic universe principle; and three novels by Virginia Woolf.

Where is it?

I find that collecting/hoarding can also lead to even more problems with organizing myself and my anxiety when I can't find what I need. What I need is very often something that I really don't need at all. But when I realize I can't lay my hands on it, then it becomes vital and doing any other task is impossible until it is found.

I was allowed to have a very messy bedroom as a child. My sisters would say it was because I was 'the boy child' and therefore could do anything I wanted (some truth). Fortunately, even if I could have done anything I wanted, I generally just wanted to stay in my room alone and read comics over and over again. It is a strange quirk that I both needed as much mental stimulation and educational novelty to be able to maintain interest and attention, yet I would also read the same comic over and over and over again (I still do).

My bedroom floor was layered, sometimes three or four deep, with old copies of *Look and Learn*, *Starburst* magazine, and horror movie books. It was a slippery surface of facts about the Roman Empire and *Tales from the Crypt*. To get into bed, I would have to jump from the door to the mattress. This way of living continued until I was into my thirties and moved into a flat with my wife. She finds security in order rather than disorder.

Though it looks untidy, I feel that mess was actually my protection. The author Joanne Limburg, who is autistic and has also written about her OCD, told me: 'My stuff is my nesting material. I don't go to pristine writing retreats because I can't write in them – I feel exposed and disoriented.'

Comedian and writer Joanna Neary, who you met earlier, cannot pack lightly. She carries armfuls of stuff wherever she goes, which she puts down partly to the horror of boredom.

> *'Even if I am only away for forty-eight hours, I will usually take seven or eight books, knowing my flashes of fascination flit about like a firefly. I think this may be nesting material too, the ability to create a Bonsai version of your world in any situation. The bag explodes open on the hotel bed and the room is immediately your space.'*

Ox-steak-guzzling guru Jordan B. Peterson has sold millions of books based on advice such as 'clean up your room'. There are those who are in a perpetual state of inaction unless everything is tidy to perfection, and many have nodded sagely at his wise words. But on the flip-side, disorder is not always a sign of unhappiness and being lost. In the hope of picking up a few of JBP's lifestyle sales, let me say:

HOARDING, COLLECTING AND OBSESSIONS

MESS UP YOUR ROOM.

NORMALLY WEIRD AND WEIRDLY NORMAL

Or rather, create a room that is in the state you are comfortable in without kowtowing to the presumed norms of tidiness. I think the past me may have battled against the physical chaos I created around me, but now I am more comfortable, as I know it represents the excitement of creativity. If you ever find yourself in Edinburgh, go to the Scottish National Gallery of Modern Art where the artist Sir Eduardo Paolozzi's studio has been reconstructed. You will see a seemingly chaotic and yet splendidly fertile space for creativity. Only clean your room if its tidiness will create the mulch to grow from, but not if it is because you think that is what should be done.

There is an Institute for Challenging Disorganization, though I think it might be more of a business model than a philanthropic venture. If only there was a helpline for the chronically messy, but if there was, you wouldn't be able to find where you had written down the number and then you wouldn't be able to find your phone.

There are however levels of mess, and it is thanks to Barry Yourgrau, author of *Mess: One Man's Struggle to Clean up His House and His Act*, that I have discovered that I am a 'clutterbug' rather than a 'hoarder'. The fundamental difference between cluttering and hoarding, according to Yourgrau, is that a clutterbug can, with great pain and emotional turmoil, get rid of things; the hoarder cannot.[7] He explains that the emotional connection of the objects to a hoarder is too great to dispose of those objects. There is a heightened 'sensitivity and imagination' around the objects. I find that the moment something comes into my possession, an emotional connection is made. Every possession becomes possessed like a mysterious charm, but I have still managed to make the leap and throw some things away.

Some may turn to Marie Kondo, the multi-million-copy bestselling Japanese author of books about decluttering, but her method does not work for everyone. Lolo, another ADHDer, told me, 'Kondo asks, "Does it spark joy?" That question is completely redundant. Yes, of course it does, that's why I own it!' I am sure Kondo is fine for people

HOARDING, COLLECTING AND OBSESSIONS

who merely 'accrue', but once I have brought anything into my house, it is imbued with emotional connections. If someone gives me a book that I know I will never read, I cannot go off and donate it to the charity shop after what I might consider to be a suitable time period after the gifting. It is immediately tangled up in the emotional framework of the giver. It might just be from someone I had never met before who came to a show and thought I might like a present, but giving it away would seem like an act of betrayal. What if they ever found out? What if it ends up in the shop window?

For a clutterbug such as me, when I realize my room is teetering on the brink of inaccessible, I will peruse and ponder at length everything that goes into the donation box.

The general difference between obsessions in people with ADHD and in autistic people is the longevity of the fascination, though this is not always the case. The National Autistic Society (NAS) quote an autistic teen who says, 'My mind was constantly whirring with thoughts, worries and concerns. The time spent with my intense interest was the only time in which I had a clear mind – it gave me that much sought-after relaxation.'[8] The NAS asks:

> When is it a hobby and when is it an obsession?
> How much autonomy does the person have to stop?
> Does the interest limit social opportunities?
> Does it create significant negative impact on those around them?

Matty told me about their mother. There was significant emotional impact. They were traumatized by their ADD mother mouldering in her five-bed house 'full of shit she couldn't take care of'. Matty knows that is in them too. They are vicious about 'stuff' nowadays. 'I threw about 90 per cent of my stuff out about ten years ago and kept only the most bare minimum.' Matty now has a 'one in, one out' policy with exceptions for work-related items.

NORMALLY WEIRD AND WEIRDLY NORMAL

'I don't miss any of the things I threw away and I feel so much lighter and less stressed by my environment. The mental load of all this shit is not to be underestimated. It's the same in the kitchen – two plates, two bowls, two sets of knives and forks – and if anyone comes over, they bring their own. No more washing-up, no more clutter, so much free brain space. Recommend it to all people with ADHD. I never looked back.'

I sometimes imagine I could be Matty, but then I begin touching the things that need to go, and they enchant me all over again.

The only time I managed to get rid of a vast amount of stuff was not because I'd read Marie Kondo, but because of a flood of sewage. One thousand LPs, books and film posters were destroyed. Twenty years later, you might think I would still be mourning each one, and yet the sense of loss and the emotional ties loosened very quickly. There was a reason they had to go. They were sodden and smelly and rotting. Nothing could be done (we tried – it didn't go well). I really would recommend, to everyone reading this: don't live above a drainage grate in an area with antique sewers near a chip shop which illegally pours its used fat down the sink thus clogging up the pipes. I have to admit, that is not as catchy as Clean Up Your Room, so hats off to JBP.

The consolations of obsessions – finding your tribe

WARNING: The next sentence may discombobulate many people in my age bracket.

I don't like the film *The Breakfast Club*. It's a film that undoubtedly helps people of a certain age imagine their life as a series of freeze-frame moments of victory under goalposts with Simple Minds playing 'Don't You Forget About Me'. It is a staple of my generation, but for me, it breaks an important rule of life. It is an insider outsider movie, as most Hollywood teen movies usually are. The nerds are

HOARDING, COLLECTING AND OBSESSIONS

always really beautiful people. The ugly duckling could appear on the cover of *Vogue* before she even takes her glasses off. But this was not the main reason I didn't like it. It is because the film suggests that you should cure people of being goths.

Ally Sheedy is an interesting introvert in a dark jumper who really doesn't put the effort in with her skincare regime. Don't worry, by the end of the film she is dressed in white with apricot scrubbed skin, an acceptable beauty. Ally Sheedy is the nearest character in the movie to someone with a neurodivergent mind, but the message is that all it takes to be happily typical is a makeover.

In my *The Breakfast Club,* she is not 'cured', she contaminates all the others with gothdom and Emilio Estevez repeatedly hollers 'release the BATS!' before there's a slo-mo shot of them all leaping up on tombstones while Nick Cave and the Bad Seeds' *From Her to Eternity* plays in the background.

When you are a social outsider and you know you cannot fit in, relief can come in the form of finding the right obsession. I wasn't a goth. I regret it now. I did have a magnificent quiff that sadly I left on a pillow one day and now my dome shines with skin not lacquer. Many neurodivergent people I know were or are goths. Far from being miserable, I have found goth gatherings such as the weekender in Whitby to be pretty happy places.

Tamsyn, who is autistic, told me she was a goth from the age of sixteen. She would sneak into the goth nights at The Racehorse pub in Northampton with her goth friend. They barely spoke to anyone, 'but it was like being in a room of fantastical creatures'. She felt a deep sense of calm and of being home that she didn't get anywhere else. 'I was ginger, specky, autistic and mostly silent so easy pickings at the senior girls' school. Goth probably saved my life,' is how she sees it now.

Danielle discovered the goth scene in her late teens. She found that there was a strong acceptance of people building a new character and life for themselves and that there was some fantasy and artistry involved 'in creating a version of yourself then taking an active part in the art and media that you consume'. She believes that the licence to reconstruct an identity through the filter of a shared culture appeals to certain neurodivergent people. 'It's generally a very creative, playful and accepting cultural scene.' Leah was out five nights a week when she found goth. She found it 'absolutely heavenly . . . All through school I'd been a fat, nerdy, specky girl and then I discovered contact lenses, eyeliner and cider and black . . . roughly in that order'.

Goth is not the only scene where people feel they could crack out of the chrysalis they had surrounded themselves with before they experienced the freedom to develop into who they really are. There is punk, metal, emo . . . Certain music tribes seem to have more 'I am not as you are' than others, as well as giving people a chance to discover a new wardrobe, easing the passage for the personality to emerge.

I have often found the more brutal the music, the more sweet-natured the fans can be. Within the fury of the mosh pit at a thrash metal gig, among the damp flesh collisions, there is real concern for each other. And I have met some very kind Satanists.

Here be dragons (and dungeons too)

The attraction of *Dungeons & Dragons* and other role-playing games among neurodivergent people is pretty much a cliché, but it does hold true and there is a good reason why. These adventures allow you to create a world and then sit and ruminate over the rules that exist within that world. Joel Morris describes *D&D* manuals as being 'like the machine code for Tolkien. It is a computer program in paper form'. If you struggle with the unwritten, seemingly arbitrary rules of one world, here you have a world where the rules are written down and specific. Everyone shares the same handbook.

Eliza Peak, a member of the Queensland Youth Parliament

HOARDING, COLLECTING AND OBSESSIONS

Programme, wrote an essay on 'The positive impacts playing Dungeons and Dragons has on mental health, particularly for people who are autistic'. These positive impacts included learning how to make decisions, learning about collaboration, and creating characters that can help break down the barriers when making conversation. Eliza sums it up:

> *'DND is a good game for all, particularly those in the autism community as it helps them connect with others and just be themselves, it is simple and easy to play so there is no way to do it wrong. DND is also inclusive for everyone, no matter who you are no one will be judged because they are playing as a character not themselves so they can just escape to another reality and have fun with new or old friends.'* [9]

Meg Leach wrote an article titled 'How Autism Powers My D&D'.[10]

> *'In my world, there are flumphs that speak with gestures and colors instead of words. Owlbear guardians travel with inexperienced adventurers, and people can evict spiders from their homes with smooth negotiation tactics. It's a world inherently amicable to someone interested in social justice, art, and mythical creatures.'*

Meg describes themself as a non-binary autistic person with many so-called quirks. They carry a notebook for sketching, drawing and writing thoughts they don't feel safe sharing. *D&D* is a place where they can feel comfortable, adventurous and use their imagination. Their first *D&D* character was 'a halfling death cleric with a mummified squirrel as a familiar. Charisma was her lowest stat, and I loved that she was more comfortable talking to dead people than her friends in the party. Her social weaknesses were vital to her character and served as a place where I could find meaning for my own awkwardness'.

NORMALLY WEIRD AND WEIRDLY NORMAL

Sadly, *Dungeons & Dragons* was never for me, as I crumble and crack when rules are read out. I can't take them in and my head spins like a Tasmanian devil. If there are more than seven rules you need to grasp before you can at least get a game started, then I am straight back to playing UNO.

The Doctor

Doctor Who has often been a safe place for the neurodivergent, even if we have had to hide behind the sofa every now and again. It also has a big LGBT following. It is a Time and Relative Dimension in Safe Space.

I have been obsessed by *Doctor Who*. I still consider the original theme tune to be one of the greatest musical works of all time and find it hard to stop myself breaking out into an excited (and obviously exciting) dance when I hear it, especially if it is a mix of every variation on the theme between 1963 and 2023, though I do take a breath during the 1980s when the uncanny influence of Delia Derbyshire got lost in the excitement that electronic keyboards were available in the supermarket. Under producer Russell T. Davies, the series has become even more flamboyant in the way it says to those who feel alienated, 'Come in and meet some aliens you will get on with!'

Online, there are many *Doctor Who* fans who ponder whether the Doctor himself is neurodivergent. Karen Clark, a teacher and sister of the tenth Doctor, David Tennant, has said that she has been struck by the role *Doctor Who* plays in people's lives and how obsessive they become, 'particularly some of the young people on the autistic spectrum . . . they know every single fact about the show . . . *Doctor Who* is such an inspiration to them'.[11] It is perhaps the maverick nature of the Doctor that appeals, the fact that they fled Gallifrey because they couldn't understand why the ability to travel time was not used to help other beings. It is the Doctor's questioning of all dogma with a mind that keeps saying, 'but why is it this way, why

HOARDING, COLLECTING AND OBSESSIONS

can't it be another way that is better for all?' that fits well into a neurodivergent framework. While maverick personalities may find fitting in the world as it is difficult, their fictional counterparts fit surprisingly well into being lead characters on television. Here I am thinking of characters such as Columbo, Monk, House, of *The Prisoner* . . . 'I will not make any deals with you. I've resigned. I will not be pushed, filed, stamped, indexed, briefed, debriefed or numbered. My life is my own.'*

I believe the continued love of these characters is because they are so much more than just brave action figures, and that it is their quirks that are their strength and their appeal.

Horror

My first happy obsession, the one that got me through my childhood, was with the dark arts. My dad and I both collected skulls found in woodlands and recently ploughed fields. My dad collected them because of his fascination with the natural world, while I collected mine to put on the little table by my bed and wait for the goblins. On that table, you would find a sheep's skull with a red candle melted into it, just as you might see on the cover of a paperback anthology of black magic stories. I never called upon Satan, but I had the props ready, just in case I needed their help.†

I was drawn to horror when I was eight years old. I wasn't scared by it and instead loved its freaks and madmen, ghouls and snake people. It was a natural thing to be drawn to when you are 'not one of the normal' – you are always cheering for the outsider, you see Quasimodo in yourself, and you wish that when the full moon was high you could turn into a ravenous man-dog creature and devour

---

* Patrick McGoohan's speech in the opening titles of *The Prisoner* (1967).
† I am presuming that Satan is non-binary. The devil doesn't seem to be one of those traditionalists who believes everything is either/or.

NORMALLY WEIRD AND WEIRDLY NORMAL

the boy who took your lunch money and threw your satchel over the fence into the bull's field. Many years later, perhaps unsurprisingly, I realized just how many neurodivergent people are keen fans of horror movies. My neurodivergent friend Johnny appears in this book incognito, and horror films have been very important to both of us in navigating the world. Unsurprisingly, when I asked him to sum this up, instead he drew a cartoon about ghosts with ADHD.

I am now a regular at the Abertoir Horror Festival, a yearly celebration of horror movies in Aberystwyth (winner of the best festival title pun twenty years in a row). When I arrived at Abertoir for the first time, I felt like an outsider. The people were welcoming, but even in a gathering of outsiders, you are waiting to be rejected. Maybe I was not outside enough? I was an insider outsider and they were outsider outsiders. What if there were a few trick questions about who designed Elsa Lanchester's hair in *Bride of Frankenstein* or who composed the music for *Hands of the Ripper* and the outsider outsiders would all know that I was not one of them?*

On the day of my show, I might have even appeared stand-offish, but really, I was just anticipating that reckoning. I stood on a stage littered with old movie mags, horror comics, stacks of ghostly novels and posters for films. My mind played ball and went into overdrive, buzzing with super excitement about all things horror, and afterwards, I knew and they knew I was one of them.

Our obsessions can cause chaos. But our obsessions also create camaraderie. More often than not, I find the passionately obsessed enjoy talking to other passionately obsessed people even if they don't share the same obsessions. There is a joy in spending time with people who are unashamed about sharing their joy and curiosity about a world others may find quite impenetrable.

---

* Obviously I know the answers to those questions, but only the other day I forgot who played Frankenstein's monster in the 1910 silent movie version. I crumbled under pressure. (It was Charles Ogle.)

7. POLITICS AND KINDNESS

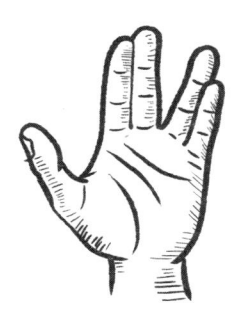

Have I killed again?

If I read about a chainsaw slaying within commuting distance from my house, a flicker of electricity in my brain creates a brief spike of worry that it might have been me. There is no logic to such a thought and there is no possibility it was me and it is soon quashed, but it is a peculiar display of neuroticism. It may be linked to the perpetual sense that I am bound to have done something wrong, and if I haven't left the fridge door open overnight or flooded the bathroom, perhaps I went on a killing spree with a chainsaw I don't even own.

Neurodivergents are particularly good at carrying around a continual sense of guilt and believing they are making life worse for the people around them, even when they have done nothing wrong at all. My emails would always begin with 'sorry to ask', 'sorry to intrude', 'sorry, it is me again', 'sorry to bother you' or maybe the whole email would be just 'SORRY'. Some days I would be saying sorry for saying sorry too much.

We commence on the back foot. As with other so-called traits, I do not think such feelings or behaviour are exclusive to the neurodivergent, but I do think it can be excessively amplified. As Charlotte said to me, 'If a stranger said ouch, even if they were 10 feet from me, I would still immediately apologize.'

One person I spoke to on the subject of guilt shared the following story.

> *'Some years ago, a young co-worker and friend took their own life, and our employers offered us some sessions with a grief counsellor.*
>
> *'Within about fifteen minutes of my first therapy session, it became apparent that I felt enormously, unreasonably, responsible for the suicide. I genuinely felt that a person I'd only spent a handful of hours with over a four-month period might not have ended their life if I had been more decisive about committing to their dinner plans.*
>
> *'It didn't require much more time with a therapist for me to see that my sense of guilt and responsibility for everything had become a lifelong habit. It was one of the most wonderful, positive things I've ever done when I learned that I am just not that powerful. What a burden to offload.'*

How wonderful if we had the power to cause such pain, because we could use it in reverse and cause miraculous healing as opposed to the humdrum reality of being at the mercy of the vagaries of the world and events within it. Annoyingly, there is no balance between taking on guilt for things you are powerless to change, and taking the praise for something helpful you have actually done.

We mercilessly search for a way to prove we are bad while frantically running away when someone wishes to thank us for doing something good. When we have saved a stranger's dog from drowning in a stormy torrent – 'Oh, it was nothing.' When we create a small chip in a plate due to a washing-up accident – 'Oh my god, I am so sorry. I must replace it at once and give you some form of financial remuneration for the psychological pain I have thrust upon you and those you love so dearly . . . There are no words to

POLITICS AND KINDNESS

express the disgrace I feel . . . I can only presume this IKEA plate was of immense emotional value to you. Perhaps it would be best if I commit hara-kiri for I have so dishonoured your crockery.'

Justice for all

Just as we spend a great deal of time in other people's minds worrying that they are judging us, so that habit leads to us dwelling on whether their cheery exterior hides their own pain. When you are used to hiding your feelings, you can't help but believe others must be too, a concern that can be for the individual or for the whole world.

Among the neurodivergent, there is often a strong sense of fairness and justice. The internal detection that leads us to often think we are letting people down, also means we spend a lot of time thinking about what is 'right'. I think part of this comes from the sense of not fitting in. If you feel awkward within a culture or society, it sharpens your focus on why things are as they are.

When you feel isolated, alone or rejected, while also covering that up as much as you can, it can heighten the empathy you feel for others. This takes me back to my frequent anxiety over whether other people are happy or content. This is not just about me worrying that I have made someone's day worse, it is also about thinking about whether I can make things better for them. Friends of Robin Williams talked of how his experience of depression inspired his drive to make other people happy, not just when he was on stage but across the rest of his life. If he saw sadness or despair, he wanted to help people out of it. He said, 'I think the saddest people always try their hardest to make people happy because they know what it's like to feel absolutely worthless and they don't want anyone else to feel like that.' Similarly, when we know how people feel on the outside, we want them to know they are not alone.

'Justice sensitivity' is described as an ADHD trait. It is defined as 'the tendency to notice and identify wrong-doing and injustice and have intense cognitive, emotional, and behavioural reactions to that injustice'.[1] Reasons given for enhanced justice sensitivity in neurodivergent people include 'emotional lability', 'emotional impulsivity' and 'negative intent attribution'. We have come across all three of these already.

> Emotional lability is rapid often exaggerated changes in mood.
> Emotional impulsivity is an increased impulsivity when in heightened states of emotion.
> And negative intent attribution is the increase in belief that intentions may be more hostile or less positive than they might actually be – a heightened suspicion of ill feeling.

Psychologist Marcy Caldwell has written that 'ADHD brains are significantly more justice-sensitive than are neurotypical brains'.[2] There is also the theory that ADHD brains 'tend to perceive information with a less positive view; this, along with cognitive rigidity and ADHD-impacted brain networks, can lead to intense rumination'. This leads to a strong need to restore justice even if it is damaging to themselves. Research by Schäfer and Kraneburg in 2012, 'The Kind Nature Behind the Unsocial Semblance: ADHD and Justice Sensitivity – A Pilot Study',[3] concluded that justice sensitivity is 'more pronounced in people with ADHD, particularly in the inattentive subtype. It is suggested that pronounced justice sensitivity may be a coping strategy for inferring appropriate social behavior.' Jillian Enright summarizes the study well in his article 'Neurodivergents: Justice Warriors'.[4] Lower levels of neurotransmitter dopamine in ADHD brains may also play their part in justice sensitivity. The mix of both minor and major injustices can be overwhelming, but the novelty of each injustice can release dopamine.

From my conversations with ADHD friends and my own experience, it is hard to screen out the discomfort of others. Things such as witnessing a child crying in the street because they have lost their

POLITICS AND KINDNESS

balloon can be nauseating, and made even worse if the parent is shouting at them that it was all their fault.

My close friend and sometime double-act partner Josie is someone who greatly helped me understand the ADHD mind. She is also a tireless campaigner and someone whose activism and passion I admire greatly. When I asked her about her first memories of having that burning sense of justice that has gone on to mark out so much of her work, she ended up telling me about her eldest daughter instead and how, from almost toddler age, she has had a burning sense of what is right.

I have seen this in her daughter myself. We were all on the way back from the local park, and Josie promised her daughter an ice lolly. Once back home though, it was realized that it was lunchtime and so the lolly was postponed. Her daughter displayed a deep sense of the wrongness of the situation. Promises had been made and then not kept. The tears that rolled down her cheeks were the tears of terrible confectionery injustice being heaped on her.

Similarly, my son was often in trouble at primary school, not for his own 'naughtiness' but for defending those who were being bullied. It made me proud to see how he sided with the maligned. On one occasion, he was being sat on by another boy in the playground who had been bullying someone else. To get him off his face, my son bit the bully on the butt cheek very hard. This finally caused him to move, and yet it was my son who got punished. I will always stand by my belief that if someone is sitting on your face as an act of oppression, then you have every right to bite them hard in the bum. This would be rule number three in my Jordan B. Peterson-style *12 Rules for Life*.

We don't know if either child is neurodivergent, but we do know that our offspring are carrying on a sense of justice which is very much part of us.* Josie's childhood inspirations were Jesus, the

---

* Next time you see me, ask about the time I stabbed a bullying boy in the cheek with an ink pen.

NORMALLY WEIRD AND WEIRDLY NORMAL

RSPCA (Royal Society for the Prevention of Cruelty to Animals) and United Colors of Benetton. In the 1990s, Benetton realized a good way to advertise was to annoy racists, so they would have billboards showing images of a black woman breastfeeding a white baby.* In 2000, their models for their adverts were US death row convicts.

Once Josie became aware of some of the problems of the world, the imbalance of power, the disparity in wealth, she could not ignore these things. She believes that the more neurotypical person may be able to compartmentalize these things, but for her, the battle to change these inequalities becomes inescapable. She also feels the intensity of the emotional tie is so strong that it can't be switched off.

Like Josie, my first memories of upset and injustice involved animals despite (or perhaps because of) being brought up in a house where my dad occasionally used to gut a rabbit in the kitchen. He would go shooting with local farmers and return with lead shot-peppered pigeons or a rabbit or, if lucky, a pheasant. One day, I think when I was about ten years old and trying to do the crossword in my mum's newspaper, I worriedly broached the subject of shooting things. I told her that I would rather not go shooting with Dad as I was worried about the animals and she said it was fine. I don't know where this empathy for fowl came from. I had similar issues with my soft toys. I would anthropomorphize them and project feelings onto the stuffing and blue plastic button eyes. You didn't have to be a living thing for me to worry about your treatment.

Atherton and Cross wrote a paper looking at why those on the autistic spectrum show an increased interest for anthropomorphism and may even show improved theory of mind.[5] They outline how those with ASD have better abilities when judging the mental states

---

* Interestingly, the outrage in the USA was from African American groups who feared the image could echo slavery. Benetton as a whole have focused on making sure they have a mixture of races in their campaigns.

of imaginary characters, and how both animals and cartoon animal characters can be easier for those with ASD to emotionally understand than other human beings.

This closeness to the anthropomorphized is beautifully illustrated by my autistic friend Jamie Knight. Most people know Jamie as 'Jamie and Lion'. Lion goes everywhere with Jamie. Lion is a four-foot-long plushie. Lion's main interests are trying to catch antelope and trying to buy Smarties in bulk. Jamie explains that Lion's origins are mostly unknown, but he is very important to Jamie and he is familiar to everyone in Jamie's life. When Jamie worked at the BBC, Lion's role was 'Antelope Manager'.

Marginalized and vilified

As I have grown older, I was increasingly drawn to the marginalized and vilified, and there were many to choose from in the 1980s – from coalminers to lesbians to black politicians and hunger strikers. Should I ever watch sport, I always want whoever is losing to win, a paradox which leaves me relentlessly without victories to celebrate.

Mairi, who runs Edinburgh's activist bookshop, Lighthouse Bookshop, is often at demos and protests. She told me that, when she sees people who look like they should comfortably fit into society and could happily avoid protest, more often than not she will find out they are neurodivergent. When I was a teenager, I was drawn to many LGBT voices, whether it was John Waters or James Baldwin. I was particularly drawn to the art of those who might be considered 'other' and who remain so. Just as I had been drawn to the stories of science fiction aliens when I was younger, I was now drawn to the undoubtedly real alienated of the Earth.

Not long before my dad died in April 2023, I was experiencing a certain level of flak with some possible professional ramifications due to a couple of comments I made in support of trans people. When I was explaining the situation to Dad, he wasn't sure why I had got involved in the first place. It certainly was true that I would have been better off keeping my mouth shut but, like Josie, often I just can't stop myself. Some of these impulses may be due to that pesky executive function of the brain again, but I must also acknowledge the role my dad played. I told my dad that day, 'It's all your fault. You taught us, through your actions, that you must treat everyone equally, that whatever their position, everyone is entitled to respect. Respect is not something to be earned, but something that can be lost.' And though I still think he was a little baffled by what made someone trans, he appreciated why I had got into trouble and why trans people deserved supportive voices. You don't have to fully understand why someone is who they are to offer them support.

Vulcanism?

Hopefully, the past decade has seen changes in the understanding of autism, but there can still be a presumption that those with autistic minds are emotionally disconnected, cold and self-centred, with an emotionally Vulcan approach to others. In a feature for the British Psychological Society on the myths and reality of autism, Michelle Duncan, mother of an autistic child, who was then diagnosed herself, explained that she understood why people might get the wrong impression and think autistic people are uncaring as she is not an outwardly emotional person. But she goes on to say, 'I help other people to the extent that it's a detriment to myself. And actually, one of the most common features of autistic people is that they have an innate sense of justice – they can't stand to see injustice around them, even if it's not directed at them.' What may appear to be aloofness due to a social sensitivity and awkwardness, does not mean that a strong sense of fairness won't exist. Indeed, tension can often arise, not from the failure to connect with injustice, but the difficulty in disconnecting from it. It can be very hard to 'just let it go'.

POLITICS AND KINDNESS

Perhaps, for both ADHD and ASD, it can be summed up as an 'intensity of feeling'. Many of us just can't let things go, however much it is troubling our minds.

Clinical psychologist Sharon Saline has written, 'Kids with ADHD tend to have a strong sense of justice, sensitivity, and of course, energy. When they feel wronged, disempowered, or unheard, they can become quite mad.'[6] As hard as we might try to bottle it up as adults, the pressure builds up until the cork flies across the room.

In her article 'Black & White Thinking in Autistic Children: Practical Strategies for Parents', Dr Lucy Russell writes, 'Autistic people often have a strong sense of justice, fairness and loyalty which is enhanced by their black and white thinking.'[7] This sense of justice is further magnified by the neurodivergent being less likely to be swayed by peer pressure and more likely to stand up for what they believe in. If someone jumps a queue, this will trigger a profound sense of injustice. She sees one of the social problems with this as being the inability to let go of the perceived injustice and this can strain personal relationships.

One of the most powerful activist voices of the twenty-first century is Greta Thunberg, who is autistic. She has developed her passion for the environment and married it with her strong sense of justice and trying to do what is right for others and the world, to become the world's leading environmental campaigner and figurehead. In an interview in *The Guardian*, she explained how many autistic people have a special interest that they can sit and do for an eternity without getting bored.

> *'It's a very useful thing sometimes. Autism can be something that holds you back, but if you get to the right circumstance, if you are around the right people, if you get the adaptations that you need and you feel you have a purpose, then it can be something you can use for good. And I think that I'm doing that now.'*[8]

She is also adept at running rings around elderly world leaders and manliness coaches when they try to mock her. Her reply on social media to sex trafficking suspect Andrew Tate after he posted that he would like to send her photographs of his gas-guzzling cars was a simple, 'Yes, please do enlighten me. Email me at smalldickenergy@getalife.com.' As the author of *Men Explain Things to Me*, Rebecca Solnit, wrote, 'She burned the macho guy to a crisp in nine words.'[9]

Emma Gorowski, late-diagnosed autistic, wrote about neurodivergence and fairness on her blog explaining that her strong sense of justice was one of her favourite autistic traits.

> 'Many autistics are fantastic social justice advocates. But our appreciation for this trait sometimes leads people into "Aspie supremacy" type thinking, where we believe we are innately more moral than neurotypicals, or to overlook the flaws that do exist in this way of thinking about and viewing our morals.'[10]

She worries that the 'black and white thinking' that may come with autism can make it hard to be persuaded out of a position. Even this, I think, has its advantages. If you know that you have an innate tendency to see things in black or white, then hopefully that awareness can lead to working very hard, as Emma does, in trying to comprehend the grey areas. I see this as one of the advantages of having had a 'problematic' mind, the need to analyse how it works and why we do what we do.

It's all my fault

An autistic friend, Paul, tells me that, if someone is annoyed with him, he automatically assumes it's his fault. He acknowledges that sometimes it is, but he has found that feeling like it's your fault all the time can lead to others taking advantage. He has been in abusive relationships, but he has only realized once he had an outside perspective. During the relationship, he assumed it was all his fault. He concludes, 'Is it any wonder that statistically the most vulnerable group open to abuse is the disabled/neurodivergent community.' This guilt can create a terrible imbalance in a relationship, handing all the power to a partner, and all the weakness and blame on to you. This negative force in a relationship can be exhausting and damaging.

Steve wonders if the exaggerated guilt he feels is because autistic people like him don't have a good understanding of what others are thinking and feeling, and so they wrongly assume negative reactions to what they do, or the intensity of such reactions. Could his guilt be a failure to accurately empathize with others, assuming suffering when there isn't much or any?

Heather has spent her life working in the health service and has felt afraid for almost forty years. A consultant psychologist who was her clinical supervisor always offered her the opening of 'how is Heather's culpa today?' If a new war started in the world, the therapist would ask her if she blamed herself. He knew that even such distant and global tragedy wasn't beyond her sense of guilt and self-blame. The predilection to find fault in yourself is the manure guilt grows in.

According to psychiatrist William Dodson, ADHD children receive 20,000 more negative messages by the age of ten than the average child. We might argue over the precise number, but just as with not having a precise number for the stars in our galaxy, we can agree that it is lots (in the case of our galaxy, somewhere between 200 billion and 400 billion). And it is not merely the disproportionate number of reprimands, but also the intensity of feeling that may accompany them. For most of my life, if I did something wrong or that I perceived was wrong, I would feel physically sick, often for days on end.

NORMALLY WEIRD AND WEIRDLY NORMAL

You really haven't thought it through

Some of my family are particularly sensitive to jokes that involve them. Like many families, I grew up in a home environment of constant banter, where mild taking the piss was a way of communicating because it was safer than saying 'I love you'. As with friendships, where some people may let banter just run off them (though probably not as many people as we might imagine), those whose minds are in a perpetual state of self-analysis can go on many journeys while trying to work out what someone 'really means'.

I have to put up a special extra barricade of censorship when I am with them so that the little person in my head who usually fails to act quick enough to prevent my foot disappearing into my mouth is extra alert. It works . . . sometimes.

The problem is that other people who speak carefully and with intention find it hard to believe that I didn't really mean something when it did just spill out as my mind made a series of rapid connections and I literally spoke without thinking. Not everything is a Freudian slip.*

I have often been incredibly apologetic in such situations, but I also battle against saying sorry all the time. There are times when big apologies are necessary but difficult, particularly the ones needed or expected in relationships. But if you are neurodivergent, you can spend a long time trying to work out the right way of saying sorry, and so a minor tiff can rapidly expand to kraken-like proportions. A little joke at the wrong time can become a dominant obsession for weeks on end, and just as it's waning, it might be given new life when you bump into someone who might have witnessed your shame.

For the world at large, there is perhaps a great deal to be learned

---

* Research actually suggests very little, if anything, is a Freudian slip.

POLITICS AND KINDNESS

from those people who don't feel that they fit in; because when you don't fit, it creates a drive for change, and it is likely to be a change that most people will benefit from. Probably, the only ones who won't benefit will be the ones who cry the loudest that a fairer society is 'so unfair!' and fear that the power they have built on the anxiety and oppression they create will slip through their fingers.

8. LOVE AND OTHER CATASTROPHES

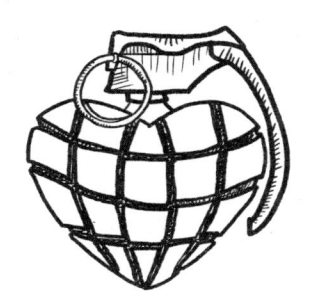

If I manage to be truly honest in this chapter, my wife will nod all the way through it and then close the book and say, 'Quite correct, you are a nightmare.' This is my attempt to understand love and relationships, which for me is up there with understanding human consciousness in terms of its inscrutability.

For a long time, I never believed that I would ever date anyone. Whatever the apparent signs of interest, however much one part of my mind would say, 'No, I really think that person does like me,' negativity dominated every other space in my head and would be laughing its head off (a head within a head) at the notion that anyone would ever be interested in me.

I attempted my first date when I was eighteen years old. I don't remember what burst of confidence gave me the ability to say yes to her invite and to go for a drink, just the two of us. It was the autumn of 1987, and we sat in the corner of the pub and listened to Nina Simone's 'My Baby Just Cares for Me' and George Harrison's 'Got My Mind Set on You' over and over again on the jukebox and conversation flowed like concrete.

It was not an awful date. It just wasn't a date because I had no idea what to do and the conversation shrivelled and died between us. I don't think she would have known that an eighteen-year-old man could be so clueless. She probably ended up assuming either that I was gay – as I wrote earlier, my taste in literature and films was very LGBT friendly at the time – or that I simply had no interest in her. It was not because I feared women; I was hugely comfortable with women. That was one of the problems. I believed that I was trusted by women as a non-threatening friend, so any presumption of romantic interest would be a terrible betrayal. The idea that anyone would have the slightest amorous interest in me was both madcap and presumptuous. I would remain unkissed as I went into my twenties.

On occasions, when sleeping on a floor of a female friend, I would sometimes be invited to share a single bed and would nervously teeter on the edge, a fall to the floor always imminent, for fear that I would accidentally overstep the mark by the error of physical contact in my sleep. I became someone who thought they would always be a great friend of women and live as a bachelor, tweedy and surrounded by tragic romantic novels, eventually dying from a paper cut after a hasty page turn in the middle of *Far from the Madding Crowd* or *The Go-Between*.

Even though most balanced minds can be disordered in the realm of romance, for the neurodivergent, in a life of heightened and sometimes rabid emotions, it's not easy to deal with that most vital of feelings – love.

Why partner?

Many neurodivergent people, out of their own wishes and sometimes necessity, can be very comfortable being alone. For people who seem quite well-suited, even happy, to be alone, the idea of partnership in life can seem a little eccentric. This does not mean that you may not want to have a partner, but you may not behave in the manner in which many expect a partner to behave.

I believe one of the major problems that can come from romantic relationships where one person is neurodivergent is that the other person doesn't feel wanted enough. Many neurodivergent people have a surprising level of self-reliance in terms of psychological needs. They are happy to be in the relationship and they wish to remain in it, but have no neat answer to 'Why do you need me?' or indeed 'Do you need me?' Self-reliance doesn't mean you want to be alone, but it can mean you are frustrating when someone wants to feel needed.

It can be very important to make sure someone else is happy, but you can seem overly sanguine in terms of what you need to take from others. This can also be within the sexual relationship too. The focus of attention becomes the other person, not you. Neurotypical people can find this strange. 'But I want to please you?' As with most things in the human sexual world though, there is a vast spectrum of sexual possibilities – so do not rely on this as your alibi to be very lazy in bed with your ADHD or autistic partner. 'But Robin Ince told me that you'd be happy if you did all the work and I just lay here in blissful reverie!'

Leslie Sickels, a clinical social worker who specializes in working with neurodiverse couples, warns that 'Without a firm understanding of how neurodevelopmental differences are coming up in a partnership, couples can sometimes believe their partners do not have the best intentions for them or the relationship' and that differences in neurodevelopment can result in varying needs in intimacy and sex within a partnership.[1]

Sex therapist Rachel Needle has written about some of the differences in sexual relationships with someone who is ASD, particularly arising out of sensory sensitivities. These differences in sensory processing can be in the form of preferences, aversions, and overall discomfort when partners are attempting intimate encounters.[2] She explains that 'as many as 80 percent of individuals on the autism spectrum have a hypo- or hypersensitivity to touch, sounds, smells, or pressure. They may become overwhelmed by arousal or stimulation and may seem to shut down or avoid sexual experiences'.

More broadly with neurodivergence, she sees that sexual problems arise when 'one or both partners end up feeling unloved, undesired, or unappreciated or when the sexual activity has become non-existent or mechanical and disconnected'. She stresses the importance, however you define your mind, 'to cultivate a safe and non-judgmental environment that fosters emotional vulnerability and encourages open dialogue about and recognition of feelings'.[3] Being in love is when we can be at our most vulnerable, and those who have struggled to mask what they see as their vulnerabilities may be excessively sensitive in any situation where they are not in full control.

I thought I would get the sex bit out of the way at the top of the chapter. There is much more that could be written, but this is the first time I have written about sex since I wrote an essay on the Christian romance novel *The Sign of the Speculum* back in 2009. It is a novel warning of the danger of attempting to have a romantic relationship with your gynaecologist. If you want to know more about sex, you can check the internet – apparently, they've got loads of stuff on it there, and it's illustrated too.

First approaches

To declare romantic interest is one of the greatest fears of being human – to be rejected destroys, which is both very silly and very serious. Every night out can be a torment of *what if, what if, what if?* followed by lying in your bedroom thinking *I should have, I should have, I should have*. There is an agony of watching the rituals which people perform, how close they get to saying 'will you?' and then the last-minute failure.

This is weird for almost everyone, our lamentable fear that brings so much unhappiness. The fear of rejection, the shame of someone saying 'thank you, but no' is so traumatic that it is better to stay silent and unloved, lonely but 'in control'. To be rejected is seen as a loss of power and control, but how much power and control do you have if you stay silent when you are so desperate to do the alternative?

For ASD people (and I would say most neurodivergent people), the ability to imagine every embarrassment and failure is a finely tuned ability. Flirting and dating are rarely easy for anyone, however confident we are. Autistic and ADHD sex educator Milly Evans has written about some of the issues when it comes to flirting between and with autistic people. Given that so often flirting is about reading between the lines of messy and ambiguous body language and verbal cues, imagine how much more confusing it can be to those of us who are autistic. She explains that it is difficult to recognize when you are being flirted with or to flirt intentionally, as sometimes autistic people are perceived as flirting when they're only trying to be friendly.

It is through her work that I discovered 'penguin pebbling'. This is a neurodivergent way of sharing with someone that you've thought about them and care about them, by the giving of interesting objects, maybe a leaf or a pebble or a shell. This is based on observed penguin behaviour, and I think it's a very sweet idea and absolutely should be adopted by everyone. It's certainly far more clear-cut than trying to observe whether the person you're talking to is touching their hair a lot, or maintaining eye contact longer than usual. After all, what is 'usual'?

She also writes about the problem of info-dumping. This is conversational behaviour frequently seen from both autistic and ADHD people where we become incredibly excited to share ideas that enthral us. This behaviour is heightened by nervousness, excitement or uncertainty about what to say, so obviously, this is likely to increase when on a date. Milly writes about how those on the receiving end can accept people's need to info-dump, but also how those info-dumping can allow themselves space to pause and ask questions of the other person in the room. The most important thing is being clear in how you express yourself, which can be particularly problematic when on a date, as the anxiety that surrounds these rituals can be subtle and confusing.

In an online article entitled 'I'm Autistic Which Makes Dating Impossible for Me', Josefina, an autistic Chilean academic based in London, who has remained single throughout her twenties, explains how she sees dating as not built for neurodivergent people.[4] She had a boyfriend in her first year at university who was four years older than her and very controlling.

> 'He got me into doing acid tabs and MDMA with him, locked in his room . . . He wouldn't really let me sleep in my own room even though it was right next to his . . . I had to ask friends from another college to help me break up with him as I was legitimately very scared.'

With the burden of not being able to detect nuance and the subtle codes that can go with communication in a relationship, Josefina felt lost. Her story also contains another ugly side of a world not structured for neurodivergent minds, her autism was weaponized against her.

The inability to be honest, the disempowering rules of the social dance can weaken many people, however their mind is structured. We need to empower ourselves with positive honesty. Too many people are caught in debilitating relationships – this is one of humanity's weirdnesses, that the cycle just keeps going.

Any system used to make people feel like they are shit people and deserving of oppression and abuse is one that needs dismantling.

While trawling about for stories of first dates in the neurodivergent world, I stumbled upon a blog post by an ASD writer who had met a man on a dating app who seemed just right for him. He imagined it would be impossible, but this man was 'cute, eloquent, and capable of substantial conversation without the drudgery of small talk. He neither subjected me to insipid messages about the weather nor his love for naps. He didn't even make me want to give him my entire savings just to get him to shut up, which is my reaction to most people'. He asked for advice from friends and felt that the most useful advice was to fight the unconscious urge to mask. Instead, he should put all his weird and eccentric flaws and idiosyncrasies out there from the start. His friend explained why, saying the dating pool is smaller for autistics, because ASD people have very specific criteria for potential partners and 'very specific needs to keep us happy . . . there are not so many people who will love, respect, and appreciate all of our differences and disability . . . [so] telling the whole truth in your most creative and charming authenticity at the beginning is a winning formula for a delightfully divergent relationship'.[5]

And I would say that that is good advice for everyone.

But now for love

What then of romantic relationships and love? What of the problems when neurotypical and neurodivergent meet and fall in love? In a world of volcanic eruptions of emotion, with the prefrontal cortex's unruly grip on our emotions, romantic relationships may face challenges.

I was lucky in my twenties to fall in love with someone on the same evening that I'd sung a cover version of the Adam Ant song 'Never Trust a Man (With Egg on His Face)'. That was thirty years ago. Fortunately, my wife didn't see me performing the Adam Ant cover, and egg-wise, I think our relationship has been bolstered by my excellence at making Sunday morning omelettes. For most of the duration of that relationship, I didn't really understand how my mind worked, and neither did my wife. Since my diagnosis, I have thought a great deal about what problems arose in my relationship with my wife because neither of us understood what my mind was doing. This ability to understand each other, to have some sense of how the other's mind functions, is an issue in all relationships, but this can be made much harder when there is an expectation that human minds should be working in a particular way and any deviation from that just needs to be trained to work correctly.

The naturalist Chris Packham wrote that most relationships he had been in broke around the five- to seven-year mark, but he believes that, with age and understanding of himself, he is now in a relationship that should last. Charlotte is his partner of seventeen years.

> 'I can't love Charlotte 99.9%. That doesn't exist in my world. I can only offer Charlotte 100% of myself – or 0%. The 100% commitment, which has previously been suffocating in relationships, is something which I hope gives Charlotte a degree of security.'

The previous relationships reached their full term because he was dealing socially with his neurodivergence, but not dealing with it at home: 'I couldn't let my guard down and that was always very challenging for my partners.'[6] Charlotte explains that Chris didn't tell her he was autistic for the first three years of their relationship because he thought he would be able to mask his condition.

> 'That's not how it felt to me though, and I don't think I handled the relationship very well until I knew about his diagnosis. I used to get even more upset about things than I sometimes do now because I had no way of explaining them.'

I can find it quite remarkable that I am in the same relationship I was in when I was twenty-three, especially when I think back to some of the intensely dark moments that we went through without any framework for explanation.

LOVE AND OTHER CATASTROPHES

Your problem partner

Now I've explained over these pages how sensitive my wiring is to shifting into total overload, how chaotic and seemingly irrational my thinking can be . . . imagine sharing a house with an animal like that.

Imagine . . .

> You find your partner has left the keys in the door overnight.
> You find your partner has flooded your flat by forgetting they left the bath running – that cupboard door being left open seems small bananas now.
> You find a piece of toast half-eaten on the armchair because your partner got distracted by a thought on atomic behaviour halfway through eating it.
> Your partner left the fridge door open before leaving for a four-day trip and all the food has rotted.
> Your partner regularly forgets to pass on important messages.
> Your partner forgot to pay the electricity bill.
> Your partner often doesn't understand something you said that you thought was quite self-explanatory.
> Your partner makes plans at 100 miles an hour and thinks you completely understood something and gets angry and frustrated when you just wanted them to slow down and spend more time explaining.
> Your partner just won't stop talking.
> Your partner just doesn't talk enough.
> Your partner bombards you with seemingly random questions while you're trying to watch TV.
> Your partner is working 2,000 miles away and rings you up to share a brilliant idea for a show they have had while forgetting it was your anniversary/birthday.
> Your partner forgot your name.

NORMALLY WEIRD AND WEIRDLY NORMAL

Tick as many as are applicable.

As you can also probably imagine, such behaviour can lead to arguments, especially because you're sure you closed the fridge door, paid that gas bill, and your partner of five years really had said their name was Joey on that first date.

For me, I think constantly living on the extreme edges of emotional breakdown has been the greatest battle.

Meltdown!

Before we cruise into the tunnel of love, here's a brief guide to the meltdowns that have plagued my life and my relationships. I have far fewer meltdowns now, but a big one happened when writing this book.

I sent off a few chapters a little too early to my editor, so that they would at least know I was actually doing something and not just frittering away my advance hang-gliding in the south of France before faking my death and changing my name. Obviously, there were faults. I write at a breakneck speed and then look at the bags of cement I have poured out and work out how to make them into something with structure, so of course, there was feedback. Perhaps because the writing had also been emotionally intense, and I had explored and written things I had kept hidden for most of my life, the first hint of negativity floored me.

By negativity, I mean something akin to 'I think we should talk a bit about the structure' or 'we're not sure about the chapter order'. But what I heard was, 'We are all very disappointed and angry. This is absolutely unworkable and some of us wish you were dead. We should never have taken on this burden of a book. We hate you and you are a disgrace!' The words weren't quite that clear, but the sickening emotions that came with them were.

I threw my arms up in the air, presumed everything I had written was malodorous and rotten, and started working out how best to pay back the advance and cancel everything. I had not had a reaction like this for some time. I had grown so used to having a healthier mind that I had forgotten how intense the sense of failure and surrender is when a meltdown hits.

These emotional meltdowns are an intense fusion of feelings of failure and frustration. The mind has no time to collate and organize or seek reason, too much circuitry is going off all at once and no one is there to control it due to that shoddy executive function apparatus that just doesn't seem to be up to scratch. The incoherence of that executive function is what makes your bedroom messy, but it also makes your emotions messy, manifesting in crying, anger, self-harm, binge eating and emotional withdrawal.

The link between self-harm and ADHD has led to a call for girls attending Accident and Emergency facilities presenting with self-harm to be screened for ADHD. In a study from 2021 on 'Self-harm as the first presentation of attention deficit hyperactivity disorder in adolescents', there was a speculative conclusion that 'Emotional dysphoria plays a role in the evolution of self-harm in dysregulated ADHD'. This led to a recommendation for 'clinicians assessing adolescents who have self-harmed to be aware of possible ADHD symptoms and screen as appropriate; however, future research examining the temporal association between ADHD, emotional dysregulation and self-harm is required to establish causal direction'.[7]

My self-harm has never gone any further than the banal banging of my head in frustration, as if striking the damn thing to make it work better. 'I hate my brain!' which translates as 'I hate me!' I used to have such meltdowns on an almost daily basis, and my wife used to find my head-smacking quite distressing. I don't think it ever managed to shift the blockage or get the motor running more effectively. When the emotions come rolling in, I have often thought isolation to be the best option, the retreat from conflict. I have joked on stage that I have spent most of my home life living in the attic like a gender reversal of *Jane Eyre*, but it is true, I *am* the madman in the attic.

NORMALLY WEIRD AND WEIRDLY NORMAL

I am not sure what the greatest problem has been in my relationship, but I would imagine the meltdowns might be a major element. I can appear to be emotionally stoical. As I mentioned earlier, my wife has seen me cry twice in thirty-two years. I wasn't happy about it on either occasion – nor was she – and it was such an unusual occurrence. There is a possible third time, when I discovered a friend had suddenly died of meningoencephalitis, but I think she was looking in the other direction.*

It can be very hard for those who are closest to you to deal with your rage or melancholy that can stem from what they see as only minor issues that seem so very slight. Once, many years ago, the basement flat I lived in with my wife had flooded with excrement and ruined hundreds of my books and records. I was in the middle of performing a month-long run of a poorly received show. I had just found that a script I had spent three weeks working on had somehow been deleted from my computer and I had to start again. A cheque I was expecting to tide us over had been lost in the post. I went into meltdown, and such was my despair, I threw myself to the floor, literally gnashing and wailing. My wife's response? 'Just get over yourself!' I had no conscious wish to roll around on the floor. I was a grown man and knew full well that this was a childish and ineffectual gesture, but the emotional overload in my mind at that moment and the inability to create a pathway to reason left me helpless. It is no fun for anyone, so I have learned that, often, withdrawal is the only option.

Sometimes a meltdown is loud and sometimes it is silent. It was the first Christmas after the first lockdown and Trent Burton (my producer) and I, as ambitious as ever, decided to do a twenty-four-hour live online science variety show from midday to midday with an all-star line-up of guests. I would be the fizzy energy of it all and Trent was going to be the slow burn who actually made sure it was

---

* His name was Christopher Price, a quite brilliant TV presenter.

broadcast and guests were where they should be. He was responsible for *everything* beyond my showing off, basically.

Trent had not been out of his flat for some time because of the pandemic and, in all the excitement of going outdoors and seeing the sky, he managed to fracture his ankle as he stepped out of the door. He hobbled around with ambitious purpose as we broadcast conversations with astronauts, songs from comedians, monologues from astrophysicists in the Antarctic, and a set from Robert Smith of The Cure. It ended up being twenty-five hours long and we managed to communicate with people in every one of the seven continents, though we didn't quite manage to go extraterrestrial and chat with the International Space Station. At 1 p.m. on day two, we bid farewell to the audience and sat in the green room eating Fruit 'n Fibre and drinking Malbec, not normally the best of pairings, but when you've been up for thirty-two hours, it works surprisingly well – the taste of success *and* digestive health.

I went to sleep and returned home the next morning. Walking through the door, I was cheered by my family. All was good in the world for another four minutes thirty-three seconds. Then my wife moaned at me for putting my bag down in the wrong place and that was that – THE CRASH. Something about her tone of voice flipped me.

My emotional radar had detected the tiniest bit of annoyance and disappointment in me in her voice and had amplified it to eleven.

So I ran.

First, I went up to my attic, mentally paralysed, deeply frustrated, desperate to flee. Sickened. I lay under a sheet in the darkness, then set my alarm for 5 a.m. I needed be out of the house before anyone was up so that there would be no human contact, no possibility for further criticism from the outside, only from within me. To some of you, I am quite sure this sounds utterly ridiculous. It sounds pretty silly to me too. But some of you will have experienced something very similar – a light reprimand with a harsh tone and then you are floored into introspective intensity.

NORMALLY WEIRD AND WEIRDLY NORMAL

Anger is an energy, but like electricity, it can illuminate, and it can send you flying across the room, twitching and reeking of charred clothing. I have spent far too much of my life being angry. First comes the anxiety, then comes the frustration, then comes the anger, often all in a little under two seconds. Most of the anger was concealed inside my head, or at least I imagined it was, but others may be better judges.

While I have always worked hard to conceal the emotions fizzing around inside my brain, anger was undoubtedly the hardest emotion to conceal. Living in near perpetual frustration and anxiety is intense physical exercise. When the anger has revealed itself over the years, I've ended up directing it at the inanimate, not the living I am glad to say. Even at my most angry, the only living thing I have ever wanted to hit is me, and I have. But doors, printers, walls, and annoying plastic things that didn't obey me as I tried to open them have all seen me at my worst.

Some anger has come from the chaos I have created in my surroundings. Some anger erupted from wider sources, such as being stuck on a train, late for an event, stationary in a field of cows. Some anger has come from feelings of powerlessness and confusion, especially in relationships. Things that I have no control over can be overwhelming.

Anger issues are not part of the diagnostic criteria of ADHD or ADD, but they are most definitely a companion of many people with ADHD or ADD. In a child, these will often be defined as tantrums, and in an adult, they will be called anger issues. Both can be disturbing for the sufferer and the onlookers and can increase that person's sense of being a no-good failure. The problem is that, by the time you realize that you have lost grip of the reins, the horse is wild. Then you get caught up in both being angry and being angry that you are angry. The anger that you have lost your temper, usually goes on for far longer than the initial burst of fury.

LOVE AND OTHER CATASTROPHES

I have read about how the best solution in the moment is to try to find your mind again by taking large breaths and focusing on your breathing, on removing yourself from whatever situation is causing you the upset (difficult on a stalled train admittedly), and in the longer term, taking up physical activities such as running or swimming, so that presumably you can cut off from such anger and focus on something more real. But rage makes reason hard to find and instructions hard to follow.

I think the number one rule should be 'learn how you work'. I think the lack of comprehension people have as to why they are feeling a certain way is part of the explosion itself. During prefrontal cortex fireworks, language can break down, and it can almost seem like we are returning to some primeval emotional rawness. We've all seen toddlers exhibit such behaviour – that misunderstanding and pain about being in the world. As we get older, we may still find that we do not always understand each other and the world around us and the inability to communicate comprehensibly with others can still bring on anger driven by frustration.

In *Irritability in ADHD: Associations with depression liability*, a 2017 study of 696 children with ADHD showed that 91 per cent of those examined had at least one symptom of irritability connected to anxiety and/or depression.[8]

The anger I regret most is what my son has experienced. I have very rarely allowed my anger to be directed towards him, but I have been short-tempered around him. I can replay the specific episodes in my mind, and they are memories where my shame is so intense that it can bring on feelings of nausea. I think the nausea is heightened because I feel that sickness in my stomach from when my father was angry with me, and I fear my son is experiencing that too. My deep memory of my childhood misdemeanours and how I was punished for them makes me particularly alert to possibilities of my son feeling that fear and anguish.

NORMALLY WEIRD AND WEIRDLY NORMAL

Don't be such a child

Chloé Hayden, actor and author of *Different, Not Less*, was diagnosed with autism at thirteen and ADHD at twenty-two.[9] She wrote of the taboo of the meltdown and how it is branded toddler behaviour, and so the older you become, the more forbidden it is. She explains how this gives those who are 'dealing with it, that struggle with it, a sense of insecurity, and discomfort, more than we're already made to feel . . . So here we go, if no one else is going to discuss it, I will. I'm twenty-years-old, and melt downs are still a part of my life. *(And that's okay)*'.

She tells her own story of attachment to objects and how that can be emotionally intense. She cannot sell books because she has memories attached to each page, she sees a ratty old soft toy deer in a charity shop and cannot bear to leave it there for fear it will end up in the garbage, and she has four pieces of jewellery which she 'loves more than life itself'. One of these pieces of jewellery is a heart-shaped ring her parents gave her when she was thirteen years old. When she was thirteen, her life was very difficult and she had been to ten different schools within a year. It is the ring that says to her, 'no matter what you're going through, no matter how hard you're struggling, you're loved'. After a day on the beach, in her late teens, she found the ring had gone. This led to what she thinks was the biggest meltdown of her life. In a blog post, she tried to put the feelings she had into words but knew that the words would not do anywhere near justice to the strength of emotions she was experiencing.

'It feels like your head is imploding, over, and over, and over again,' she writes. 'You're stuck inside a volcanic eruption. Inside a nightmare that's repeating the *jump-scare* section of it over, and over, and over again. And it's really, really scary. Because it feels like, in the moment, there's nothing in the world that can bring you back out of it.' She explains that this is why anyone with sensory processing issues and 'anything else that stops our systems from running with our senses *regularly*, often hit themselves, rock, scream, or cry when they're in melt-down-mode'. As her ability to comprehend diminishes, that sense of shutting down has gone so far that Chloé has even passed out.

On the occasion of the lost ring, when her dad asked if her 'pity party was over', she went straight onto social media, drenched in snot, and asked whether anyone had a metal detector. The ring was found. She uses the events of that day to remind herself that pity and sorrow and falling into a heap does nothing.

> *'Get up, wipe away your snot and your tears, and try. The end result may not be what you want, but you're never going to know unless you try. And hey . . . Having faith the size of a mustard seed, can help you find something equally as small.'*

Suicide ideation

At 5.10 a.m., the morning after the meltdown I had when my wife complained about my bag, I left the house as planned, silently, and walked in the winter dark along the frozen canal to an unheated shared office space I used occasionally at the back of an old town building. It was ripe for haunting. No one would be in for at least four hours.

My brain was too stuck to read or to write, so I just moved things about, feeling the anguish circulating around me, pointlessly tidying a pile of stuff that was really beyond repair. I went home eventually, but it began a three-month period where, if my wife asked me, 'What are you thinking?' I would reply, 'Nothing in particular,' or 'The disappointment of the *Robocop* sequels,' when I was actually thinking what I would look like hanging under a bridge. The ultimate escape fantasy.

Suicide ideation is a daydream that many people have experienced, though few act upon. This is the fantasy of forever silence – imagine just not having to deal with this confusion and pain. Beckett wrote, '. . . you can't go on. I must go on. I'll go on.' Anthony Newley said, 'Stop the world – I want to get off.' Somewhere in this fantasy of silence lurks the knowledge that you could not enjoy your fantasy as the fantasy requires you to cease to exist.

Though my suicide ideation stemmed from feelings of hopelessness and sadness, I think it was different from the strong suicidal intent that can come with depression. It was driven more by the need for silence than the need for total termination. There was a sense of self in it that I believe is absent from many of those who attempt to or succeed in taking their own life. When I have spoken to people who have tried to take their own life, they have expressed a sense that, at that lowest point, the themness of them, that sense of self, of being someone, was almost entirely gone.

In 2017, the Centers for Disease Control and Prevention believed there were approximately 10 million people in the USA who experienced suicidal thoughts. In that year, there were 1.4 million attempts of suicide, and it is estimated that only 2–3 per cent of those who experience suicide ideation will die by taking their own life. In the paper, the authors state there is little understanding about the transition from suicidal ideation to suicide attempt.[10] Like so much in mental health, the first barrier that needs lifting seems to be our ability to discuss what lies within. Suicidal thoughts should not be a dirty secret.

Research has shown increased depression and suicide ideation in college students with ADHD,[11] and also a significant rise in suicidal ideation in women with ADHD but not men.[12]* There is a belief that the link between ADHD and suicide ideation is made stronger by the

---

* As hypothesized, the association between ADHD symptoms and suicide ideation was accounted for by stress, and this effect was strongest at high levels of stress-reactive rumination.

increased levels of stress experienced due to ADHD. The ideation can seem heroic or vengeful. When I was thinking about suicide in boarding school, it very much had a feel of 'that will show the bullying bastards'. Then I realized that it probably wouldn't and I might screw it up and anyway it was double English tomorrow and we were doing *Picnic at Hanging Rock* which I really enjoyed. It does not have the desperation and utter loss of connection that comes with true suicidal urges, though you can never be quite so sure when you are in the midst of the fog.*

A 2014 study found that anecdotal reports supported the idea of increased rates of suicidal ideation in adults with Asperger's syndrome (now ASD), and that depression is 'an important potential risk factor for suicidality in adults with this condition. Because adults with Asperger's syndrome often have many risk factors for secondary depression (e.g. social isolation or exclusion, and unemployment), our findings emphasize the need for appropriate service planning and support to reduce risk in this clinical group'.[13]

The Royal College of Psychiatrists highlighted the case of Daniel Willgoss, who took his own life when he was twenty-five years old. In a presentation titled 'Suicide and Autism, a National Crisis', his mother, Sue, now an adviser on suicide prevention for an NHS foundation, highlights statistics that include autistic adults with no learning disability are nine times more likely to die by suicide than the general population and that it is the second leading cause of death among autistic people. Recommendations to tackle this include improved diagnosis of autistic people and ensuring that mental health services are aware of the increased risk. Ways of support include believing the autistic person who tells you that they feel suicidal, 'even if such information comes in a different or unexpected manner', and listening.

---

* I am skipping over this a bit as I wrote more lengthily about it in *I'm a Joke and So Are You* (Atlantic Books, 2018).

NORMALLY WEIRD AND WEIRDLY NORMAL

As a child, anger and despair came easy to me, and they continued to do so, and it is only since my diagnosis and the medication I now take that they seem to have receded somewhat. I haven't experienced suicide ideation since I spoke to Jamie about my mind and my emotions in 2022. It was one of the things that was vaporized by coming to an understanding about myself. It was gone before the anti-anxiety medication kicked in. I realize now that the most annoying thing about these dull fantasies, these illusions of being Thomas Chatterton, were how much space they took up. It meant my head was playing the same movie over and over again, when it could have been playing with something far more interesting.

I am lucky that I can enjoy this new bandwidth and that it lets me be creative rather than destructive. Though the local plasterers are less pleased now they don't get as much work from filling in the holes in my walls.

9. COUCH or HOW I MET ME

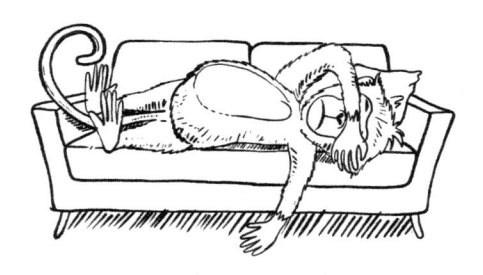

Sam, who is autistic, told me, 'Self-knowledge is a hell of an effective medication.' Knowing thyself is not as easy as it sounds. Even though you hang around with you all the time, a day can still come when you realize that you are not who you thought you were. Some people are so worried about meeting themselves that they avoid it at all costs and spend a lot of time in the pub instead.

I did.

Therapy

I found myself in therapy just before I turned fifty. I had been interviewing therapists for a book I was working on. At some point during each interview, the therapist would say something like, 'I presume you're in therapy, Robin.' I would smile and say no and their faces would drop into bafflement and their eyes would say, *oh dear, I think there has been an oversight.*

What I saw as the indulgence of therapy had never seemed like an option to me. It felt too much like showing off and I was already showing off on a nightly basis, shouldn't that suffice? I had a family and a career, despite the anxiety and self-hatred I felt and despite the chaos that accompanied me. Fortunately, I had become friends with a therapist called Josh. We first met at a book festival where we shared a breakfast table with a confident man who wished to tell us many stories of his time working on *Beverly Hills 90210*, a show neither of us had ever seen, although I'd once seen someone vomiting on leading cast member Jason Priestley in a London pub. Being Canadian, he took it very well.

Josh was one of those people who I instantly knew I shared common ground with, not merely due to our lack of knowledge of 1990s teen soap sensations, and it was Josh who encouraged me to risk a little therapy. He would have been the perfect therapist for me, except by then it was too late. We had become friends, and this muddies the waters of therapy. He said that Samuel Beckett used to go drinking with his therapist. Perhaps that is why his work seems to get more and more miserable with age, though I am thankful he didn't become too happy-go-lucky. The stranger-ness of the act of therapy is an important part of it. It is through our lack of attachment in any other way that we are able to reveal our secrets.

Josh explained that, from the first time we met, he had a sense that I was battling with something. I thought my carapace was watertight and opaque, but clearly it wasn't. He summarized it for me.

> 'Without knowing exactly what it was you were struggling with, I just had a sense that you were struggling, and that it would be good for you to go somewhere where you could just play that out. I will say to people, sometimes, "well, maybe a bit of counselling would be better," or, you know, even rarely, if it's a very specific symptom, like fear of flying, "so maybe you need to try a bit of CBT". But it seems to me that a bit of analytically oriented work would help you because the main thing is just that someone speak freely, and feel that you're being listened to, without judgement or agenda.'

COUCH or HOW I MET ME

I had often been wary about how many therapists seemed to be charlatans, with their little bronze plaques by their doorbells, seeing the world through such a particular prism that they will insist on persuading you that your problem is whatever theirs is or what they are writing their next book on. Before you know it, after a month on the couch, you're overly obsessed by the burden of a memory of falling into a pile of monkey poo in the baboon enclosure at London Zoo as a two-year-old and how this is why, when you see any of the colours of the mandrill monkey, you are triggered into deep psychosis and constipation. Only later, after a conversation with your mother and by finding a less baboon-obsessed therapist, will you discover the whole thing was built around a false memory implanted in you, but by then you are swinging in a tyre and hurling your faeces at window cleaners and bike couriers.

That said, on my fourth birthday, I was hit on the head by a ball that a dolphin was playing with at Windsor Safari Park, and I then got trapped in a rotating gate at the exit. Ever since, I have always panicked if anyone kicks a ball near me while I am walking through a park, and I've been very sheepish about going on playing fields. Should I blame the dolphin?

Being able to go to a therapist is not something most people have the luxury of. In England and Wales, it's a long journey to get to the point where you can have access to a therapist within the health service. Then you are just assigned someone and it is a lottery as to whether an effective relationship will arise.

My friend and collaborator Trent, who has suffered from anxiety and depression for much of his life, first had therapy in 2001. For him, as for many others, there is an issue of time constraints. The current system gives you anywhere between six and fourteen weeks of therapy, and then it is time to move on. With one therapist, he had a strong feeling of an imminent breakthrough, but there were only two more sessions left. He remembers the therapist apologizing for being unable to continue. Trent asked if he could re-enrol and wait his turn. She explained the system just didn't work that way. When his time came, he would be assigned someone else. He knew that the progress made would fragment and disintegrate over six months and then he would have to start all over again. Eventually, he found a way of getting discounted private therapy with someone but discovered after about seven sessions that the therapist was deeply Christian. They were casually trying to convert him, which wasn't really Trent's thing.

He remembers the therapist saying, 'Imagine one morning you woke up and you'd experienced a miracle. What would you do? How would you react?'

He replied, 'I would go "What's this?" and try to work out what actually happened that meant something looked like a miracle.'

The therapist said, 'That's your anxiety trying to rationalize it. This is just a miracle.'

The back and forth continued and Trent's refusal to accept a miracle confirmed the termination of that particular therapeutic relationship. Trent believes in the remarkable; he just doesn't believe in the miraculous. Perhaps if he witnessed some lepers being cured by the touch of a bearded man in a smock he might be persuaded, but even then, he'd want to know that this messiah wasn't slipping those on the receiving end dapsone with rifampicin (and maybe a little clofazimine too).*

Being lucky enough to have a therapist choosing my therapist for me, I wanted to know why Josh picked the therapist he did. He explained that a lot of people choose a therapist with whom they can take refuge in a reinforced version of very disciplined rules over a very long period of time, but he reckoned that would not be for me. He was right – rigidity rarely suits me, as I relentlessly pick at the seams of any sack someone tries to put me in and wrestle with

---

* These are the current antibiotics used for Hansen's disease, which used to be known as leprosy.

COUCH or HOW I MET ME

any title I may give myself, like a fevered dreaming man fighting with his blankets.

Josh believed I would need someone who was not so austere. The person he suggested, he thought, came across as an ordinary human being, with the capacity to show how she felt about things. He felt she could manage human exchanges in their full range and wouldn't feel the need to rein things in, while still having a good boundaried practice. Ultimately, he hoped that I would enjoy it, and the therapist would too.

When the therapy began, unsurprisingly I realized I wasn't very good at it. I worried too much. All the anxiety of talking about the anxiety got in the way of me expressing the anxiety, and in the early stages, I don't think I even realized how dominant anxiety was in the problems I was experiencing. I have spent much of my life being anxious about not upsetting people. It makes me deeply unhappy to make other people unhappy (though I do occasionally make exceptions for my enemies), and this now included my therapist.

My mind would move rapidly to check anything I was about to utter and see whether it was going to bewilder or annoy or cast me as a rancid pervert in the mind of the listening therapist. 'Don't say that, she'll think you are a narcissist/a misogynist/masochist/sadist...' pretty much any -ist except harpist or optometrist. Perhaps you need a special therapist if you are someone who worries about pleasing their therapist.

Mute with anxiety, I would lie on my therapist's couch in silence staring at the wallpaper. Fortunately, she had interesting wallpaper. I think it was Dutch. It had windmills and labourers by a river. About twenty minutes in, I might rapidly say something and sigh, then return to being silent. For the last ten minutes, I was so worried that I would accidentally go over time and annoy my therapist that I would remain silent again, ready for a prompt departure.

More obvious signs of anxiety were that I would always ask to use her loo before the session and afterwards. I would worry that

NORMALLY WEIRD AND WEIRDLY NORMAL

I would suddenly be bursting to go to the toilet once on the couch, but too nervous to break the session and ask to use the loo, so I would lie in silence with an agonized bladder.* On the way out, I would worry that I would get 100 metres from her house then realize I needed to go to the loo, and have to return to her house, blushing, asking to use the loo and then be confronted by her next patient. Perhaps this patient would even be my mother (who died five years earlier).

When I did begin to talk more coherently to my therapist, I became overly concerned about being repetitive. Much like a regular stand-up gig, I presumed I should always deliver as much new material as possible, as talking about the same old thing would mean I was being lazy and she'd pick me up on it. 'Oh hell, I did that stuff about my dad's anger last week, I'd better improvise something about my mum's depression this week.' She would tell me that it really was fine to go over the same stories, but I felt that was what a hack patient would do. 'Don't bore your therapist' became my pointless mantra.

Worrying about my therapist

I also worried about my therapist. I wanted to ask how she was. She was slim, and when I heard her stomach rumbling, I would silently wonder if she was eating enough and start to obsess about whether she was happy. I wondered whether I should bring in cereal bars and then leave them by the cushions of the chaise-longue . . . or bring soup. I make good soup.

When I told Josh about this, he said, 'That is proper transference.' Transference is when you project feelings you have in general or about someone else onto your therapist. It made sense. If someone

---

* It was etiquette and a full bladder that killed the astronomer Tycho Brahe, and he had a nose made of gold. If he couldn't excuse himself, who can?

COUCH OR HOW I MET ME

wants to know how I am, I am always far more worried about how they are.

> *At this point of writing, I am worrying about you. I am worried that this is not useful enough to you and may be way too self-indulgent. Suffice to say, I hope you are doing okay and we reach a point where this chapter is mutually beneficial.*

I had of course researched my therapist online and I found out that her husband had died young. Whenever I started to broach anything about mortality or loss, not wanting to upset her, my mind would hastily turn it into being about something else. I believed I had been brilliantly discreet, that no one would EVER have known that I had been about to talk about death. But she was smart, or I was stupid, probably both, and she saw through what I was doing, and one day she stopped the session and said, 'It is not unusual to look up your therapist on the internet . . .' And she went on to explain that I shouldn't shy away from the subject of death, that she was dealing with her own grief and I mustn't think talking about grief was out of bounds. But of course, all that happened was that I worked much harder to hide it and updated the early warning software of my brain.

My other issue was trust. Deep down, I had a mortal fear of trusting anyone with my innermost thoughts, of letting anything out from the safety of my uncomfortable mind to where it might be used against me, the sort of thing you hear the Scientologists do. 'Tell us everything about yourself, every fault and hushed desire. Excellent, we have that on tape, now you can never leave.' Once a thought is freed, once it has broken out of the safety of the prison of your brain, who knows where it might go.

Even revealing my socks became an issue. On the first day, I was told it was okay to keep my shoes on when lying on the couch. This meant I had to make a choice, to keep them on or take them off. As you know by now, no decision is simple, everything for me is a choose your own adventure game with multiple possibilities and the imagined outrages that go with them. Would she think I was rude for keeping them on? If I took them off, were my socks okay? Did I have a hole in them, having forgotten it was a Tuesday? Should I buy slip-ons to visit my therapist, so that I wasn't wasting time fiddling about with difficult footwear? How would I be judged for being someone who wore slip-ons?

Weighing up the different levels of possible shame, I went with keeping my shoes on and tried to avoid mud and puddles on the journey there. Flip-flops would have been the easiest option, but I have ugly toes and odd nails. And what does wearing flip-flops say?

I imagined a group of therapists drinking together and laughing at their idiot clients and their shoe and sock habits.

'You should see the socks one of mine has, they don't even match.'

'One of mine got dog shit on the scatter cushion the other day while he was holding the Jungian truth bowl.'*

From an early age, I have lacked trust. I didn't even trust my mother to support me in the swimming pool when I was trying to learn front crawl. It wasn't so much that I didn't trust my mum, or felt that she had a secret desire to drown me, it was just that I knew things could go wrong and, even wearing armbands, my mind would race to the possibility of my own death. I didn't trust the person holding the abseil rope when I went on an outward-bound course. Instead, I stood trembling at the edge of the rockface and became a laughing stock. For many years, I didn't trust zookeepers to adequately secure baboon enclosures either, and dolphins are definitely a no-no, however much they tell me that it's going to be okay.

Therapy wasn't all wasted wallpaper time. We did get somewhere.

---

* I should make clear that I have no idea what a Jungian truth bowl is. I do not think it exists, but in my dream, it is full of petals and they went everywhere, but I would like to make it clear to the Freudians that there were no teenage nudes in my vision like in *American Beauty*.

COUCH or HOW I MET ME

I realized that what I saw as a multitude of different issues, from irritable bowel syndrome to self-loathing and a perpetual sense of failing others, might all be down to my anxious imagination. A myriad of concerns and spasms was really just one thing – I was always worrying about the imminent worst-case scenario. Negative thoughts are the stickiest thoughts, as they are the ones that warn us of danger, however absurd the danger might be. This was the first time I truly confronted how anxiety had dominated my life. It was a breakthrough, and this new understanding took me to the next stage, though not immediately.

'It sounds exhausting being you'

One day on the couch, after my usual ten-minute, mid-session monologue when I would run through the litany of difficulties I was having being me or even wondering if there really was a me, my therapist summed up and said, 'It sounds exhausting being you.'

I had never really thought about the exhaustion of anxiety, of continuous scrutiny. I make myself busy whenever possible, so any tiredness could be explained by a belief that it was the real deadlines and not the fantasies in my head that were the issue. But anxiety wears you down. And then anxiety doesn't just exhaust you in itself but it also refuses to let you sleep and recover, by keeping you awake at night being anxious.

As someone who had spent so long scrutinizing every one of my thoughts and feelings, I was fascinated by how my therapist could add even more levels of scrutiny. One day, when I arrived, she asked me why I had emailed her in advance to try to change an appointment time for the following week. I did not lie back on the couch, as I thought this was a practical question only requiring information, but she soon put me right. 'WHY did I feel the need to email? WHY did I want to change the time?' I lay back and began counting cart horses on the wallpaper again.

NORMALLY WEIRD AND WEIRDLY NORMAL

On another occasion, she wondered why I was also slightly late paying my bill. I thought about this. I would always leave the session, thinking, *Right, I will pay this bill for the month as soon as I am home*, and then something else would happen when I got home and my mind would run off in another direction and then the month would pass and I would miss the payment again.

I began to wonder if it was something I was subconsciously doing. After all, I knew I was the sort of person who let people down. I was bad, so my mind would, behind my back, keep putting off payment so I fulfilled the prophecy of me. Now I am aware that it was not some subconscious masochism, but instead, put it down to that easily distracted cortex that just can't concentrate. For a while though, I really came to believe that this was not distractedness, but deliberateness – the desire for punishment. It's what Freud would have wanted.

At the time of my therapy, I had not yet been diagnosed, either informally or formally, as being ADHD, and it does make me ponder whether we are missing things like ADHD in the hope of more 'traditional' psychotherapeutic interpretations. There are many reasons for this. ADHD has been presumed to be a childhood disorder that improves with age, though really it may well be the concealment of it that improves with age. When getting an official diagnosis, you need a report from someone who knew you in childhood. So the older you get before going through the diagnosis process, the fewer people you have who you can choose from. By the time I went for mine, pretty much anyone who was a good judge of me from my childhood was dead. As was pointed out in 'Misdiagnosis and missed diagnosis of adult attention deficit hyperactivity disorder', 'many clinicians are still not aware that ADHD is a valid diagnosis in adults'.[1] The paper also points out that some clinicians 'also believe that hyperactivity symptoms must be present for a diagnosis, resulting in those who present with predominantly inattentive symptoms being overlooked'.

COUCH or HOW I MET ME

Is there a me?

During the process of therapy, my unrepentant self-scrutinizing mind stumbled on a newer worry – did I exist?

I wasn't worrying that I was a ghost or merely the figment of someone else's dream, though I do worry about those things if I read too much Philip K. Dick on a hot day. Instead, I started to worry that there was no real personality or innate self, and that all that existed were my interactions and performances with and for other people. I was empty and existed only upon contact with others. I was interested to see that this subject had popped up in a chat room for autistic people.

> 'Most of my life has been an act. I have internalized multiple personas over the years, pretending to be someone I am not, regardless of whether this someone is real or a figment of my imagination. As an extreme example, once, when I was at school, I imitated the precise way a girl pouted her lip. I ended up pouting my lip and must have looked quite ridiculous.'

In another forum, the question of unstable self-image came up.

> 'Being autistic you are often exceedingly sensitive to your environment and just absorb it like blotting paper – this again is not conducive to a strong sense of self – you are impacted upon more by your surroundings/others than vice versa and can feel your actual self vanishing. My self-image goes up and down like a yo yo dependent upon who I am interacting with/around – it's very disorientating.'[2]

Similarly, there are cases of ADHD people who are constantly trying to cover up what's really going on in their minds, which can lead to becoming disconnected from a cohesive sense of self. So much time and energy can be spent trying to fit in with others that you worry you are losing who you really are behind the mask. Looking back now, with the knowledge I have gained since, I realize that being relentlessly conscious, by never going into an autopilot of social interaction, you can feel there is no instinctual self.

Fear of bringing chaos into the room

The real treat of therapy days for me, though, was its proximity to an excellent charity bookshop. I would always arrive at the station early so I could slip into the shop and buy some unnecessary books. When I got to the therapist, I would always leave the carrier bag outside the room. One day, she asked, 'Why do you always leave your bags outside the room?' and she made me realize that this was not just an innocent action. I left the bag outside the room because I didn't like bringing physical chaos in with me. If I came into her room with it, I would feel that I was messing up her room and antagonizing her. As you now know, many people with ADHD have become so used to the sense that they bring chaos that they work extra hard to try not to make a mess, though they normally create some other form of disorder in doing so.

I stopped therapy after a few months. I liked my therapist and I thought she was smart and understanding, but maybe that was the problem. Whenever I meet people I like, I want to be friends. Obeying the rules of stranger-ness took work. I would walk into the room and notice a book I knew about and start talking about that and then see her look of soft admonishment. I was not paying her to be a friend.

When I tell Josh about this, he tells me it works the other way around too. He tells me of a patient that he really liked and how he felt this was enough of a problem that he took it to supervision. He told me, 'It really drove me crazy because it was very obvious that if I had been sitting next to him at dinner, we would hit it off.' Josh explained that my worry about wanting to be friends and knowing this was not correct said something about me. 'It was about your need to take on the problem and to take responsibility for the problem and manage it yourself.' I think I have always been someone who feels the need to take responsibility, even if others wish that the job was given to someone else or would rather that I butted out.

Going to therapy also requires a rigid commitment to a schedule and, another unsurprising turn of events, I just couldn't keep to the schedule. I was back on the road touring, and my need to say yes to every gig offered to avoid letting down venues and bookers meant that my wallpaper-scrutinizing days were over. Like most of my life, I turned it into a comedy routine and moved on.

I was still some distance from knowing my own mind, but the realization of how relentless the anxiety in my life had become started something stirring. I had also started to understand the aphorism, 'people in therapy are often in therapy to deal with the people in their lives who won't go to therapy'. We can believe that we are the broken part that needs mending while entirely dismissing that some of our damage can be from the world and those around us who create obstruction and fear.

This brief trip into therapy was the beginning of me realizing that the agonies of the whole world might not be entirely my fault.

10. REVELATION OR THANK YOU UNMASKED MAN

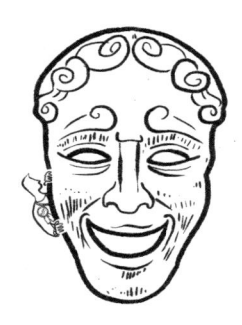

'Why fit in when you were born to stand out?' – Dr Seuss

Not long after the end of therapy came the COVID lockdowns, mismanaged for maximum damage and inconvenience by the UK government. As you may well have experienced, either with yourself or with a friend, lockdown was a period of time where many people could no longer run away from their own minds and collided forcefully with them. Many of our coping mechanisms and escape routes were closed off. The initial lockdown went okay for me. My friends and I worked out lots of ways of making online content to connect with people and it worked. We descended or ascended into busyness. In some ways, it was much easier. Real life social situations beyond those with my family were banished. So many of the usual chaotic interactions were removed, but something was still ticking and I journeyed into a dark land which seems almost otherworldly to me these days.

Much like being surprised by the letters from school that resurfaced, I was strangely relieved when I found this email that I had sent to my therapist friend Josh in July 2021.

NORMALLY WEIRD AND WEIRDLY NORMAL

Hi Josh

I hope it is not out of order asking a bit of professional advice, feel free to be abrupt or ignore.

It has been a strange time not being able to perform and it has really brought it home that being on stage is where I can let out, in some shape, form or noise, all the things that I hold in and put a mask on for the rest of the day.

One of the things I have realized is that I am driven by trying to make people happy and pretty much always believe I have failed. After conversations, interviews, shows, whatever, I always feel that I should probably say sorry, that whatever I have done is not good enough and has let people down. Even after a night out with an old friend, I will leave thinking 'Did I bore them? Was that shit? Was it a terrible night for them?'

Every now and again in stand up, I have a night where that does not happen and it is tremendous relief.

In my private life, this does not happen. I very rarely, if ever, believe I have made my wife happy. She seems cross or disappointed most of the time – you probably won't remember a joke I did at Soho theatre about catching that look in your partner's eye which seems to say 'but would I be happier as a melancholy widow?' – it is probably the truest bit of stand up I have ever performed. My head is always jam-packed with conversations I will never risk – chamber pieces of 'this is what would happen if I really answered "what are you thinking?" honestly'.

I realize that, without the usual distractions, I think about suicide a lot. I suppose I always have since quite an early age. It is very boring. I know it is ideation – is that the right word? – rather than something I would act on. I am quite

REVELATION or THANK YOU UNMASKED MAN

aware that the damage it would cause to my son and others would make it something that I must not do, plus I am probably entwined in the fail, fail again, fail better cycle of all that useless hope which will mean I keep going until my heart gives out or a vein in my brain pops.

Really, just more chamber pieces in my head.

I suppose I would just like to turn my head off for a while.

I am sorry to ask you about this, but I just wanted some advice from someone I trusted in this area.

I hope things are okay with you and I am sorry to ask about all this.

Robin

Josh was his usual helpful and compassionate self, but before we got the chance to meet and discuss it all, something happened at exactly the right time.

It began in a place of aggression and fury, Twitter, or X as it is now called. I had been addicted to Twitter for some time and it was a place where I had experienced frequent abuse, some from real narcissist bigots and others from seemingly cross bots. But I had also made friends on Twitter and learned from Twitter. My final lesson from Twitter, shortly before I departed the virtual stocks for the last time, came from an autistic stranger. I had seen an interesting account called Jamie&Lion. Their posts were thoughtful, informative and funny. Shortly after pressing the follow button, I received a DM from Jamie&Lion.

Hi Robin,

Thanks for the follow. It's a little surreal.

NORMALLY WEIRD AND WEIRDLY NORMAL

> I'm not sure what the best way to approach this chat is? Mind if I just blurt out my thoughts and then see how it goes?

I find much communication difficult, agonizing or impossible, but talking to strangers who get in contact with me out of nowhere much easier, whether face-to-face after a show or online. I said yes to Jamie right away. I was intrigued, and perhaps I already had an inkling of what it was about. The pressure in my head had been building.

Jamie replied.

> Sweet.
>
> I think it might be worth exploring the neurodivergent model a bit. The more I hear you talk, see your tweets and hear your perspective the more familiar it gets.
>
> It's something I encounter often in my work. A lot of folks who are coming across ADHD/autie stuff later in life have similar experiences.
>
> Lockdown has been exceptionally good at bringing the barriers to the fore. Another common path is for someone's kid to be diagnosed and they recognize themselves.
>
> I say lens rather than diagnoses. The medical lens is very useful, but it's often misapplied to autism the same way it was misapplied to sexuality.
>
> The ND [neurodivergent] more is about recognizing patterns and traits and the barriers we encounter. Then finding tools to engineer away the barriers.
>
> This is already very long. Trying to fit a huge topic into a single message.

REVELATION OR THANK YOU UNMASKED MAN

My reaction to this message was excitement and worry. I knew that I might finally get an answer to something that had been swirling around me and within me for so long. I was nervous – what if there was no solution, what if it changed nothing? What was interesting to me was my immediate and complete trust in a total stranger who, at the beginning of that day, I hadn't even known existed. My manic side was fully switched on and ready. The excitement trumped the anxiety. I approached this without suspicion. Though, within this bubble of excitement, I still imagined the judgement of others, in particular my family. I was staying over at my sister's. Should I tell her who I was going to be having this long Zoom call with and what it was about? Would I have enough privacy? What if someone could overhear or should burst in?

I already liked the possibilities that would come with Jamie's approach. This was not about being given a badge and then flashing it whenever you felt your failures or pain, this was about finding what you needed to navigate the world better and improve your life. The label is for you to use how you wish, but with the label comes an instruction manual.

A few days later, we set up a Zoom meeting. There was no fumbled preamble, I just started talking to this stranger with an intimacy that I had never really been able to achieve with the therapist, my family or my friends. I realize now that I was clicking with someone else with a neurodivergent mind, with rules of engagement that I could understand. As I know even better now, there is something about that connection between many neurodivergent strangers. There is an openness. There is not the threat that can occur with some of the more typical people of the world #notalltypicalpeople.

I still cannot get over the timing, but maybe I am looking at this wrong. In one way, I see it was a time where the bleak had built up again, but maybe it wasn't so much that it had grown, more that it had just gone on for so long. The obstructions were the same, but I was just so tired of it all. Sure, Jamie had contacted me at a time when the grey thoughts were getting harder to shift. I would try to drive them away by hanging out with my son, looking for LEGO pieces, and watching films about superheroes that were an hour too long (for me, but not for him). Even then, I would sometimes think, 'I wonder if my son likes me or would rather hang out with a different parent?'

But I also think this was about what began maybe sixteen years before. Initially, the change in me began with who I was as a performer, but that onstage change was really an offstage change that got its greatest chance to be exposed when in the spotlight. As the years progressed, what was happening with Jamie now, had become increasingly inevitable, and yet, had I not friended him that day on Twitter, or had he just not seen the notification, then maybe this almost inevitability could have still been missed.

Jamie asked me a series of questions about my life, some of which were about the darker thoughts I was experiencing and some of which were as simple as, 'Do you leave cupboard doors open?' To which I replied, 'I don't think I do, but my wife tells me I am quite wrong about that.' We leapt from Scandinavian melodrama to domestic banality and back again.

The banal and the mundane can often reveal really deep things about ourselves. For me, not closing the cupboard doors could often lead to blazing rows with my wife, so I paid particular attention to closing the cupboard doors, just as I paid particular attention to not flooding the bathroom (not always successfully). I was so aware of being accused of casual cupboard-door-opening that I had sometimes thought about taking photographs of closed cupboard doors, but then realized that bringing out such evidence during an argument might look facetious. Also, how would my wife know that I had not merely taken a series of closed cupboard pictures on a single day and then falsely implied that it was the day in question?

I really believed that I was cupboard competent, and this was why

REVELATION OR THANK YOU UNMASKED MAN

I would get so frustrated. The realization that these behaviours were about my inability to finish so many tasks, even something as simple as closing a door, because my ADHD mind was flying at such speed that every second there was another new thought obstructing the continuation of the previous action, was exhilarating and exciting. The priorities of the world and its realities were changing for me second by second.

Maybe I wasn't a lazy good-for-nothing?

Even the busiest and most successful neurodivergent people are very good at believing they are lazy time-wasters. They might have created a perpetual motion machine while running the London Marathon in record time and composing an orchestral extravaganza and all before lunch, but by 2.30 p.m., they will bemoan the fact that they have totally wasted yet another day and done nothing, just because they have spent an hour on TikTok watching forty-second clips of TV hospital dramas.

Discoveries like this can be hugely helpful for relationships. Many people believe, in such situations, that their partner just doesn't care about them, or their feelings, or their cupboards. When they see another open cupboard, they take it as a sign that their partner spends their life thinking, *Can't be bothered, they can close it for me*. Actually, they are thinking, *I should ring Ed. I should reply to that email about health insurance. I should write a poem about ice-skating. I should start singing Johnny Cash songs in the voice of Vincent Price. I should go and rearrange all my CDs in the order of the country of origin of the drummer*, and all those thoughts are stacked on top of each other and only the Vincent Price rendition of 'I Walk the Line' gets done before the end of the week. Neurodivergent behaviour patterns can be interpreted as a lack of respect towards the person you love.

Within the first hour of my conversation with Jamie, things were falling rapidly into place. The great fear of seeking a diagnosis is perhaps that you will discover that there is nothing there and that you are just shit, but the great transcendent moment is actually discovering that you are not shit – you are different, but not shit. The more Jamie talked, the more I knew that I had been burying all of these things for decades. Every time the reality of my mind peeked through the soil, I would hurl more dirt on top, keeping it hidden. Jamie's conversation was a universal digger which, with precision, removed all the detritus I had used to conceal what I must have known but refused to acknowledge.

As I write now, I am smiling at the memory of that conversation. Just as my emotional memory used to store everything I was ashamed of, since that day, it has become much better at recording ecstatic experiences so they can be replayed, and this is one being played right now. I am leaving my Plato's cave of scary shadows projected from my own eyes.

Jamie and I spoke a great deal about internal voices, about how we always imagined the worst-case scenario, and about how quickly one's mind makes connection after connection after connection, so that within the space of a minute, you have started nine different stories as each short pattern of thoughts creates another possibility. We talked about the rapidity of our thoughts in general, and the rarity of silence, and how annoyed we became by the noise. And then we got on to sharing the relentless sense of failure we often felt and how dismissive we were of our successes and how that would completely crash our mood. I think we spoke for three hours. It was so easy to talk.

At the end of it all, Jamie told me that all of what I had shared reflected an ADHD mindset. I don't know why this statement should have been so seismic for me, but it was. It created a crash zoom of perspective. It was as if I had been staring at a Magic Eye picture for fifty-two years, only seeing a fog of dots, and suddenly, I could clearly see a dove flying over an oak tree with every leaf and branch

REVELATION or THANK YOU UNMASKED MAN

and feather sharp and defined. It was there all the time – what had been stopping me seeing this?*

I have spoken to many whose neurodivergent diagnoses came later in life, and the two common quandaries have been, 'How did I not realize this before now?' and 'Why has this made such a seismic difference to my relationship with myself and the world around me?' I think many of us knew all along, but lived in a private world that would not allow us to confront the truth. Perhaps we exist feeling that we are bad and shabby people undeserving of anything better than what we already have. As long as others believe in this makeshift version of ourselves, then we don't need to worry about ourselves.

The shift in that understanding, which is so momentous, is something I don't think I will ever truly understand. It is why I had to write this book. There is no moment in my life that has been so utterly and positively transformative.

It all makes sense now

A pragmatic impact was the realization that the chaos of my live shows was a positive thing, not negative. My inability to be linear as a performer was not a bad thing; it was why people returned. For twenty years of touring, I had walked off stage after almost every show with a sense of failure. I have spent so much time lying in budget hotels in my hair shirt after a show thinking I had failed the audience, however many of them had laughed, cheered and wanted to buy me a drink afterwards. At 1 a.m. or 2 a.m., I would often tweet my apologies for having been so awful and disappointing to the people of Bromsgrove or Barnstaple or Balamory.

After talking to Jamie, I realized that the very thing that I

---

* Actually, I can never get the hang of Magic Eye pictures. All I ever see is dots and confusion.

thought destroyed and shamed me was actually just my creative mind at work and something to be celebrated. The audiences had not been returning to see me out of masochism. They had not come to the show in the hope that I would deliver a well-planned, linear performance with a precise narrative arc; they had been there for the chaos of ideas. The very disorder I had scolded myself for was the attraction.

I had been trying to mould my mind into an impossible shape, a shape it was not intended to be. A mind that leapt around making connections at speed – the speed to create negativity, was also the speed of creativity. Somehow, I had not been able to understand until this moment that my battle to be 'normal' was a pointless endeavour. Like our physical shape, we think we can starve ourselves or exercise our body until we reach some pinnacle of ideal, but others have different body types, different genetics, different hairlines, different bumps and biceps and whatever lies underneath, and we should not try to be them as we cannot be them. We need to find a way to be comfortable and healthy in the physical shapes or mental forms we have.

I began to realize that the propaganda of normality, sold so relentlessly, did not have to be a necessity, and the idea began to build for me that, rather than suppress what lies beneath so I could be someone else, I should fertilize my peculiarities and grow into what I truly was, and that it may well be something rather wonderful.

The actor and impressionist Rory Bremner was diagnosed with ADHD when one of his children was also diagnosed (this seems quite common). When I met him after he had found out, I thought it was odd that now he had a diagnosis he behaved as if he had ADHD. What a clot I am. It was not that he was now behaving in line with the diagnosis he had been given, but that he had spent most of his life concealing what he was and now he was happy that the concealed person could come out of hiding.

REVELATION or THANK YOU UNMASKED MAN

The question is not 'why do people gain eccentricities at the point of diagnosis?' but 'how much of a struggle was it to keep all that way of being hidden for so very long?' and 'just how much energy is drained by so many neurodivergent people working so hard to be "normal"?'

After my conversation with Jamie, I wondered if I should tell my wife. I feared that she would be annoyed with me or just think I was showing off. When I nervously told her, her face beamed. She was pleased and said, 'That would be wonderful, because I've always thought you were bipolar.'* She still thinks it is best to keep me in the attic, understandably.

Once you have been given the power to recognize yourself, you can recognize so many other people's struggles, just as Jamie recognized mine from a distance. I now wore a lens that allowed me to see other people clearly too. I realized it was likely that many of my closest and longest relationships were with people who also had neurodivergent minds.

This does not necessarily mean they have minds that behave in exactly the same way as mine, but they may have minds that do not feel as if they fit in with the wider world. Perhaps they are battling with social rules. Even if the individual battles are different, the war can be very similar.

---

* From my experience and conversations with bipolar individuals, you will likely find quite a few crossovers. Our definitions are pretty ham-fisted.

11. DIAGNOSIS – I DID, WHAT ABOUT YOU?

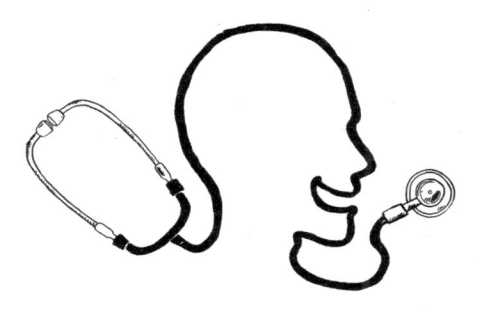

Now you've heard about my diagnosis, what about yours? Or perhaps that friend you've been concerned about?

My hope is that as various levels of neurodivergence become normalized and come into open and plain sight, more and more people won't need a diagnosis to be able to navigate the world more effectively. For now, I think a diagnosis can still be very useful for people. We are, as humans usually are, in a transitional phase of understanding.

Two diagnoses

I have experienced both an unofficial diagnosis and an official one. As you know, the unofficial diagnosis came first and was brilliantly timed. It came from out of the blue when I was in a grey zone. I was both falling and at my most open to talking. I didn't need the second official diagnosis for myself, this was for other people.

I didn't enjoy the official diagnosis and worried about it for weeks beforehand. I had gained this new understanding of myself through Jamie. What if I went into the 'official screening room' and had this new understanding of myself taken away again? I was far more comfortable being diagnosed by someone else who lived a neurodivergent existence than being scrutinized by a neurotypical expert in the field. It was probably the most anxiety I had experienced since the combination of diagnosis and medication had crushed my old worry patterns. Even when I 'passed' the official test, beyond some momentary relief, it didn't mean a great deal to me.

I obtained the official diagnosis because I knew of the cynicism towards ADHD. I had already experienced such voices from a few people I worked with and from others, though not from anyone I was close to. I thought an official badge with paperwork may help them more than me. The sense of being judged as an impostor still weighed on me too.

Some people seem driven to dismiss ADHD and many of the late-diagnosed autistic people. It's as if they consider such people a great inconvenience to both them and the world. Some react as if it is a threat: 'Oh, so you think you're more special than me!' I call this 'the vegan outrage'. Far more people bang on about vegans banging on than vegans actually bang on. There are those who believe that there is just one way things are meant to be – eating roast beef and pork scratchings, for instance. Should anyone not eat roast beef or pork scratchings, this is seen as both an affront and an attack. Those who don't drink alcohol will have found themselves similarly interrogated and scolded.

The cynical attitude of the wider world can be one of the reasons people decide against diagnosis. The persistence of negative attitudes towards neurodivergence in a crowd can heighten the sense of 'what's the point, it will just cause more trouble. Put your head down and keep going into the abyss'. A good time to remind you that sometimes you don't need to change yourself, you just need to change your friends.

I think the negative attitudes can come from envy mixed with a little fear. There's a worry that you may have found a way of escaping unhappiness, and so, you may be less sad than them and that's just NOT FAIR.

In the introduction to Gabriel Weisz Carrington's biography of his

DIAGNOSIS – I DID, WHAT ABOUT YOU?

mother, the artist and author Leonora Carrington, he writes that, 'For those who live in emotional poverty, other people's happiness is a threat'.[1] With the increase in understanding and diagnosis of neurodivergence, autism, ADHD, dyspraxia and dyslexia, there is the threat of people not merely being happy, but also being harder to manipulate. Also, as I experienced myself, you might be thinking *this is all nonsense* because you are in denial.

I know so many people who are so much happier and finding life so much less of a challenge now they have a diagnosis, whether official, unofficial or self-made. Sadly, we live in a world where critics keep saying 'Prove it!' But the more of us there are and the greater our camaraderie, the harder it will be to be dismissed.

There is also the fear of change. Things can be bad, but what if you risk a move that could lead to change and that change is worse. Many people stay in jobs they don't really like because the certainty of dissatisfaction is less risky than aiming for something better that could possibly lead to confronting failure. We can be very risk averse when it comes to our ego. I think the benefits far outweigh the risks, but the apprehensiveness is quite understandable.

At events, I am often approached by people recently diagnosed as neurodivergent and I can usually tell, because they hold themselves in a way that says, 'I carry far less sadness and self-criticism.' I particularly see this with women who have finally been diagnosed with autism in late middle age. They have lived their whole life under so much pressure and now they are confidently autistic and confidently themselves. There is far too much pressure on proving your mental turmoil. Are you hurting enough, or is this just the correct amount of pain for living?

Official help with mental health is often elusive. Sadly, the UK health system (and I expect some others) far too often waits until someone is truly and visibly broken – attempting to take their own life, for instance – before anything is done. Rather than work to avoid the breakage in the first place, we wait until someone has been shattered by their despair before we take action. If a society's priority is not finding ways to support and increase the happiness for those that live within it, then what is the point of it? If we want a healthy and successful society, we must find better ways of ensuring people are not living lives characterized by constantly frustrating and destructive internal battles.

I have heard many impassioned pleas from people on the subject of our unhealthy attitude to mental health. I was told by someone, who feels wracked with severe OCD, anxiety, phobias, agoraphobic depression and reclusion, that if she had been helped when she was seven years old and trying to look after her nan who suffered with severe manic depression, she wouldn't have spent a lifetime struggling. As an ADHD-diagnosing paediatrician told me, 'It's heartbreaking and exhausting trying to provide the service people deserve. Being told "there's no money" for a decade now is frustrating. We are working flat out to see the new people we can and keep the follow-ups going.'

Governments must understand how important mental health is. We need a system where people are unafraid to be open and have access to help. Being mentally healthy should not be viewed as a luxury. And the more we are able to be comfortable with who we are, the more we are able to reach out and help others fighting those battles. And that is another reason for camaraderie and communication. Many will be waiting far too long for official diagnoses, up to eight years sometimes, so as amateurs with personal experience, we need to be there to help people through and be guides when needed, just as Jamie was for me.

The official diagnosis

Before I went for my diagnosis, I met someone else who diagnoses others. It's good to practise.

Dr Alex Curmi is based at The Maudsley, the largest mental

DIAGNOSIS – I DID, WHAT ABOUT YOU?

health training institution in the UK. The man at reception had *love* and *hate* tattooed on his knuckles, something which I imagined might make some of those coming to deal with their anxiety a little sheepish as they approached the desk.

Alex works on diagnosing people with ADHD, thinking about which types of question are the most useful at helping to work out how people's minds function. He explained that it is often the banal aspects of everyday life, like the cupboard closing, that can be the most revealing. He told me:

> *'Ironically, a lot of stuff that has a big emotional flavour, like suicidal ideation, like self-criticism, I tend to filter out. I cover it, but it's not so diagnostically useful because lots of people have suicidal ideation and don't have ADHD. Lots of people have self-criticism.'*

He finds that a lot of the most useful questions to ask are around lack of executive regulation. These are the mental processes that enable us to plan, focus attention, remember instructions, and juggle multiple tasks, such as shutting cupboard doors. Alex shared with me the list of questions he often asks during assessments and I am pleased to note that he will now add 'cupboard door opening and failing to close' as a key indicator.

His list of questions are things such as:

Do you start something and then fail to complete it?
Do you unload half the washing machine and/or half the dishwasher, and then leave the rest?
Do you fail to finish tasks that most people would finish?
Do you need to have everything within your visual field, so that if something's not in sight, you lose memory of it?
Do you need to meticulously take notes when someone is giving you instructions?

NORMALLY WEIRD AND WEIRDLY NORMAL

> Do you feel like in your mind there's a constant, loud monologue and you can't get your mind to shut up?
>
> Do you feel that when you have less distraction that voice gets louder?
>
> At night, when you're trying to sleep, do you find yourself being relaxed by stimulation?
>
> Are you most relaxed when you're playing an intense video game?

If he has patients who have tried cocaine, he always asks how the cocaine affects them. They will often say, 'I felt relaxed and I could focus while everyone around me was partying. I didn't get it. I felt super calm for the first time.' It is not surprising, therefore, that cocaine is very chemically similar to the stimulant treatment that is used to treat ADHD.

> Do you feel a constant sense of restlessness?
>
> Do you feel frustrated by slowness?
>
> Do you feel like you're in a rush for no particular reason?
>
> Do you finish other people's sentences?
>
> Do you intrude on other people?

How did you do? I did pretty well. Though I was not there for an official test, it underlined what I had learned already from Jamie.

Not everyone needs a diagnosis. But whatever you are, neurodivergent *or* neurotypical, I think it is important to gain the new strength that can come with self-comprehension. I think it is useful for all of us to spend a little time working out why we feel as we feel and why we think the way we think.

While I was in Sydney making a show about spiders, I was approached by someone as I stood by a web, and she said, 'I think I'm ADHD too.' She wondered about being diagnosed. I asked if she was happy. She replied, 'Very much so.' So I suggested that, if she

DIAGNOSIS – I DID, WHAT ABOUT YOU?

was doing more than okay, then she probably shouldn't bother with a diagnosis. But she should just be aware of how her mind interacts with the world, be alert to why certain problems may arise, and I recommended a couple of books.

If life isn't posing too many problems for you, then maybe it isn't worth seeking a diagnosis. Equally, do not dismiss your unhappiness or confusion with life as something you just need to get on with and not bother anyone about.

Diagnosis day

When I ask people about the experience of hearing the diagnosis and how it affected them at that moment, many reflected that it felt like a great weight being lifted.

This weight may seem at its heaviest the closer it gets to the diagnosis appointment day. I found that my mind began to fill with uncertainty and the anxiety of 'what if I am wasting everyone's time?', despite my conversations with Jamie. My fight or flight system was undoubtedly really kicking in.

Having spoken to many therapists and psychologists, I have learned that very, very few people who seek a diagnosis do not have some form of neurodivergence. There seems to be an idea that many people are just casually strolling into doctors' surgeries in order to get diagnosed with a neurodivergence so they've got some kind of alibi or excuse for life. It's a theory that does not stand up to scrutiny. And yet it continues to get trotted out.

Should you ever find yourself wasting time watching a news panel show and the discussion is about any sort of mental health, then in the supposed demand for having a balance of opinions, it is highly likely that at least one panellist will have some suspicious story of how they knew an employee who claimed to have anxiety/depression/whatever just to place unbearable demands on a wealthy employer. Often the story is played for laughs. 'They said it was impossible for them to work unless they had an office with a view of the Thames/twelve tomato plants and a donkey/a machine that pumps out meteorite dust on Tuesdays.'

This mean-spirited and, I believe, predominantly fictional story-telling of the unbearable burden of these pushy people with their 'mental health issues', will sometimes take a brief pause when a well-known person takes their own life, and all of a sudden, the collective that has been making its appearance fees by mocking mental health issues starts pocketing appearance fees for asking 'why didn't anything get done sooner to help them?' instead.

From my conversations with mental health practitioners, many of those seeking diagnoses are also people with deep-seated fears of judgement, excessive social shame and anxiety, so to put yourself in front of someone who is going to 'judge' you is not a minor issue.

A friend of mine described the day she went to be diagnosed, after eighteen months of waiting and many more years of being haunted by uncertainties about herself and whether her mind was 'right' or 'wrong'.

> *'The day I went in I was scared. Convinced they would say I was making it up, that everyone does that, everyone is like that. I felt guilty for spending money on a private appointment, and a weird impostor feeling, that I was trying desperately to be labelled as something, and that surely wasn't a normal thing to do . . . Getting diagnosed with autism, ADHD and dyspraxia was . . . revelatory. Suddenly, I wasn't just stupid or broken or not good enough.'*

This was typical of the response of many people when I asked them about the day of their diagnosis.

DIAGNOSIS – I DID, WHAT ABOUT YOU?

Other people's stories

Many also talked about the outpouring of emotion they felt.

> 'I cried with relief. I'd spent so long learning more about ADHD and seeing myself in it and allowing myself to think that maybe there was an explanation for why so many things that should have been easy felt so hard.'

Many women said that they had avoided getting a diagnosis because they didn't think women were autistic. It just wasn't a possibility. One friend told me that she had to repeatedly ask to be referred for an autism diagnosis, but that in Lancashire, it was seen as an exclusively male preserve until 2010. Her response to her diagnosis was predominantly that she felt vindicated. She had waited a long time, but those closest to her had already accepted that she was more than likely on the autistic spectrum, and she was supported by them.

When I asked Kathryn, who was diagnosed with ADHD, how she felt when she was diagnosed, she replied, 'You said "how did I feel", and taking that literally and being alexithymic,* I don't have words for the feelings, even now, nearly a year later. Ironic! Probably "deeply validating" is as close as I can get to a feeling.' She went on to explain how she felt a sense of being truly seen in such a way that all her memories and past suddenly made sense.

Others had less positive experiences when they were diagnosed. For children, particularly, diagnosis can be a double-edged sword. For someone diagnosed with ASD when they were eleven it meant 'I got extra help in schools, but this also meant the other kids ridiculed me . . . They regularly called me the "R" word'. But as they got older

---

* Alexithymic – having difficulty experiencing, identifying and expressing emotions in yourself.

and started to attend sixth form college, they suddenly realized their true friends were ones who accepted them for who they were. 'After that, I not only began to accept the autism, but I embraced it!'

There can also be a sense of resentment. Judy started understanding herself more when her son was diagnosed with ASD and then ADHD. After her own diagnosis, she felt bitterness and 'a little bit of anger'. She knew she would do everything in her power to help her son live his life, but her bitterness came from wondering why no one had done that for her, why no one had noticed her enough to help. On the positive side, she now knows about masking and how exhausting it has been, and she doesn't do it as much any more. She is now proud to be who she is and does not feel the need to hide herself, and she is able to find 'her people'.

Even after the possibly preposterously long wait, not everyone has a positive experience. There are cynics in the system.

Sarah, the cosplaying Mad Hatter, visited her GP to ask about a referral to seek an autism diagnosis. The GP's reaction was 'Why? What's the point? You know they can't cure it, don't you?' This reaction was deeply unsettling and seems to have come from someone who enjoys the unfortunate status of power without the balance of understanding and humanity. Unlike many physical illnesses, the 'cure' for neurodivergence, more often than not, comes from gaining an understanding of yourself that then allows you to make your life and the lives of those around you easier. Though it seems that, when society finds a problem in people, it rarely sees changing the way it works as a solution to that problem.

Whether or not you get a diagnosis may also depend on the mental health services available to you. I was told of the frustration experienced by someone who had been greatly encouraged by their partner to seek help and the anxiety he faced as the day approached after the long wait. When the day finally came, 'he was triaged by a cold non-specialist who was literally just ticking boxes based on questions and not listening to his actual answers'. His wife

DIAGNOSIS – I DID, WHAT ABOUT YOU?

believes that, because he holds down a job, a family and a home, and doesn't memorize lists or statistics, he doesn't meet the criteria in their area's testing for autism. At the end, he was told any issues he had were something his wife should deal with. He felt utterly embarrassed and ashamed.

One of the first replies I received about diagnosis was from someone who, at twenty-two years old, had reached a point in their pain and struggle that demanded a solution. They wrote:

'Sat in front of a therapist, for suicidal thoughts and depression. Just after being made homeless, due to parental rejection, after prison for a crime I didn't commit, which resulted from an abusive relationship born out of the fact that I couldn't accept my sexuality. I already had self-worth issues from childhood, bullying for being different and trauma from being bullied for being overweight as a child and to me realizing I was gay was just the straw that broke the camel's back for my ability to accept myself.'

As they were diagnosed with what would now be termed ASD, they described the experience as being like getting 'a set of instructions to an appliance that knew it was going wrong but wasn't actually broken. It was like a light in the darkness. It wasn't just like an answer to a question, but it was like being told the question itself'.

That understanding of not being broken but being different was another oft-repeated experience during these conversations. Cade told me that they were sixteen when the possibility of being 'medically different' was raised. Cade describes themselves as 'a weird kid who struggled a lot in high school, after doing surprisingly well at primary'. They got put in detention most nights through secondary because they didn't do their homework and didn't do well with essays. Cade was kicked out of school at sixteen.

Cade describes being diagnosed with autism, ADHD and dyspraxia as a revelation. 'Suddenly, I wasn't just stupid or broken or not good enough. I'd been let down by my school because they "didn't want to label me". They made me feel stupid because they didn't want to put in the work.'

When Cade went to be assessed for dyspraxia, their mum came along too. Once in the office, she dropped her bag on the floor, spilled the contents, and then spilled her cup of tea all over everything. The assessor looked at her very sympathetically and said, 'A lot of parents discover they have similar issues as their children at these sessions.'

One reason for avoidance comes from the belief that, because other people are suffering more than you in life, it is narcissistic to seek help for yourself. Just because you know other people suffer worse things than you, it does not mean that your suffering has no meaning. To mitigate your pain because someone else is in more pain is only necessary if we are dealing with the last bottle of morphine in the medical tent. Then your sacrifice means something. (My father once told me a touching story of his father, a man I never knew directly, but I came to know from this story that kindness and fairness were qualities that ran in our family. My father said that, when his father was dying in hospital, he kept trying to refuse the oxygen as he was quite certain there must have been someone who needed it more than him.)

A diagnosis can help someone understand themselves, and consequently, it can also become easier for other people to understand them. Someone wrote to me to explain that their ADHD diagnosis had helped her, but additionally, her husband had said she had become a totally different human, which sometimes makes her feel she has been unfair to him because she is not the person who he married.

One person told me of how an ASD diagnosis had thrown them into 'a state of regret and grief for weeks'. They thought of all the situations, fun and people they had avoided previously and the opportunities they had let slip by, because they were too scared to

DIAGNOSIS – I DID, WHAT ABOUT YOU?

ask for support or feared failure or rejection. But after the grief, there came a sense of relief. Now they could 'officially' get the support that was tailored for them. They concluded, 'I'm not broken, just tuned to a different wavelength, and that, although ASD is a key influence on my behaviour, thinking and personality, not everything is a symptom. Seeing it as something to explore now, and own'.

Octavia told me that when she was diagnosed with ASD she experienced grief, especially thinking about her mother, who had died before Octavia found out about ADHD and ASD. Her mum said Octavia had a flip-top head. 'I feel like she really tried, and I feel very sad about that because she must have thought that she was just wrong. Because I was having tantrums, you know, smacking myself in the face. And then over the years of addiction.'

Though grief may well come with diagnosis, Octavia knows the diagnosis was vital. 'I wouldn't have completed the first part of the course without that, because it meant that I could have a learning studies agreement. It just opened the floodgates for understanding myself a lot more.'

It's not all about a diagnosis

An official diagnosis can of course help enormously, especially with the impostor feelings that many neurodivergent people experience as they worry that they are making everything up or are not really autistic or ADHD or depressive, so maybe they are just pretending to be deeply unhappy and/or confused in the world, just pretending so methodically that they believe it themselves. An official diagnosis is not everything either. Though a certificate from someone in an office can be a very useful confirmation for many, there are also those who come to their conclusions through their own research and that can be enough.

Kathryn is the parent of an autistic and ADHD diagnosed child, and she has become increasingly aware of her own ADHD behaviour and other family members' ASD, but she has not reached for a diagnosis, because the understanding has already been helpful and brought a level of internal peace for herself. She found the initial realization surprising. She began to understand that her friendships that work are all 'neurospicy' ones. She explained that all the friendships that have broken down, or even just fallen by the wayside over the years, are the ones where the other party was neurotypical.

The author Matt Haig, who has written extensively and usefully about his own mental health battles, went quiet on social media for a while. When he returned with a new book project, he put up a statement about his diagnosis of autism.

> *'I know some think it pointless, as an adult, to get a diagnosis of autism. After all there are no magic autism pills to take. But for me a diagnosis has changed my life. Knowing why my brain is a scramble after a busy day of meetings in London for instance helps. Once I used to escape that discomfort by heading straight to a bar to drink it away. Now I know nothing is "wrong" with me and that my mind will settle in a couple of hours. It means I stay healthy. Understanding is its own medicine.'*

I have had it easy; most have had it far harder. One respondent wrote about the power of their diagnosis:

> *'. . . the fallout from all I've been through has made life really hard and really shit. And to the present day I'm still struggling in trying to get my shit together. But that moment of being told I had Asperger Syndrome was a moment of beautiful freedom that I've been given. A moment where I realized I had my finger on the issue so at least I was facing my issue.'*

Some people experience an elation that lasts, although for some, the relief is then tempered. I was told of a person's 'blissful feeling

DIAGNOSIS – I DID, WHAT ABOUT YOU?

of pure relief' on hearing their ADHD diagnosis, partly due to the 'burning anxiety' they had experienced the previous four months while they were waiting. They felt the desperate need to have it affirmed. After a couple of weeks, they slumped into a period of sadness and struggle, as they tried to come to terms with the loss of the lives they had never had, while also experiencing the rollercoaster lurches from the search for the best medication. They concluded that it was still difficult on many levels and always will be, but they 'try to remember that profound feeling of validation because it was and is important. I believe everyone has a right to know themselves, and even if treatment isn't possible, diagnosis must be made more accessible'.

Poet Clare Ferguson-Walker was diagnosed as bipolar over twenty years ago. This was not an immediate salve for the struggles she had been experiencing, but it was the start of something. To know who she was more clearly did not instantaneously vanquish all her difficulties, but she emailed me and ended with these warrior words.

'I've spent the vast majority of my adult life trying to rewrite the negative conditioning that engrained itself into my consciousness, it's not been an easy task but as my second collection of poetry Chrysalis *is about to be published, it feels like teenage me can justifiably stick 2 fingers up to every teacher who told me my life would come to nothing.'*

She also said something that rang very true for me.

'It's taken a long time to accept it, it felt like a coat that just didn't fit properly, uncomfortable and restrictive, not to mention the fear that uttering the fact of it in social circles might send people running to the hills.'

I had been unaware of the heavy, itchy, wet coat that I had worn for so much of my life. That itchiness, that arch in my back from the weight of it . . . it just felt like it was unavoidably me. I never knew there was a way of throwing it in the bin.

Understanding, whether it is understanding yourself, other people, or the laws of the universe, gives us more power, the power to change what is wrong or unjust and a route to find comfort and joy in our existence.

Metamorphosis?

Your transformation can also transform other people. Just as they may see something new in you, you may see another side of them revealed, and it is not always a positive change, whether in the workplace or in friendship.

People get very used to who you are or who you have pretended to be. They can usually get used to a new moustache quite quickly, with some malleability depending on whether it's a pencil, Zapata or an extravagant Dali. A stealthy wig or facial tattoo can take longer, but a mind behaving in a new way can take the longest of all. Some who would be happy with you adopting a new Stalin 'tache and getting the cast of *Help! . . . It's the Hair Bear Bunch!* tattooed on your cheeks might find your new inner confidence quite impossible to stomach.

Not everyone will understand this change, and they will tell you that they were sure everything was alright before 'all this' as if they had a privileged view of the inside of your mind. Some will feel that they don't have the control over you they used to have – with new confidence comes a reduced susceptibility to being controlled and bullied. Being more comfortable in your own skin can make other people itchy.

I think my friendships that crashed on the rocks after diagnosis were those whose existence relied on my weaknesses.

DIAGNOSIS – I DID, WHAT ABOUT YOU?

Robert, who is autistic, said that, if people had liked him in general before his diagnosis, the diagnosis was helpful because he was able to explain things to them about himself that they had perhaps found tricky or complicated. But if people hadn't accepted him in the first place, 'especially if there was a falling out, then no amount of new information would put right a falling out, or someone's initial impression of me, if it was the bad one'.

After everything, I remain an insufferable human being to live with, but my wife has a framework and can now see where some of my more insufferable traits come from, and I can be more aware of my errors and how I can go about rectifying them. My increased knowledge of my own nature means I can try harder not to bring Carrie-like chaos to our house, but my telekinesis does flare up every now and again, around prom time.

12. MADDER WHEN SANE

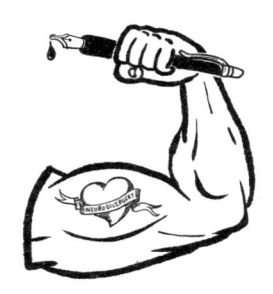

Some people seem driven to dismiss neurodivergence, particularly in late-diagnosed people. It's as if they consider such people a great inconvenience to both them and the world. Some react as if it's a threat: 'Oh, so you think you're more special than me?!'

The broadcaster and comedian Ruby Wax believes that we have still not reached a point where being honest about ourselves with others is always best. She has written numerous books about mental health and has been very open about her own battles. Back in 2016, when she was being interviewed by *The Times*, she said:

> 'When people say, "Should you tell them at work?" I say: "Are you crazy?" You have to lie. If you have someone who is physically ill, they can't fire you. They can't fire you for mental health problems but they'll say it's for another reason. Just say you have emphysema.'

More recently, in an interview in *The Guardian* promoting her book *I'm Not As Well as I Thought I Was*, she wrote, 'I've spent a lifetime creating a "front" to give the illusion that all is well. It wasn't and it isn't.'[1] Even in showbusiness, a supposed haven of the mentally flamboyant and eccentric, there is a sense that there is only so much that should be revealed, (unless you are making a documentary about your pain that has international sales potential).

Confident vulnerability

Jamie told me of a power he now possesses, and I believe that I do too. It is called confident vulnerability. Rather than your vulnerability becoming an anxiety or a driver of melancholy, you lose your shame about it, and it becomes powerful. I experienced a moment like that when I was in Glasgow talking at Mount Florida Books. It is a favourite bookshop of mine for many reasons, including the fact that the shopfront still announces itself as a tattoo parlour, and last time I visited I met a pipistrelle bat.*

I was in the midst of talking about why being able to write your thoughts down on paper can help you understand yourself and the world more. My talks are rarely planned, so I had no idea that this would lead to me talking about my mother's car crash. As I started to explain how my relationship with my childhood and with my family changed after writing about the accident, I was caught off guard by a surge of emotion. I paused, wary of becoming overwhelmed. My stomach retracted as I felt the sadness, the sense of pain that my parents experienced and the lostness of us as children, as it suddenly and vividly played out in a microsecond.

The tears hadn't yet come, but I knew if I didn't breathe a little more they would. But I was not ashamed. I was worried for the audience who may be feeling lost or unnerved. I told them that this would only be a momentary pause.

All was quiet.

Then, a man from the back, his voice intense with compassion, said loudly, 'You take as long as you need.' It was a beautiful connection, and I saw it travel around the room like a light trail left by a

---

* You can read more about that in my book *Bibliomaniac* (Atlantic, 2022).

firefly. I sensed that my story was also affecting him. So I walked to the back of the room and I hugged him and then I came back out front and continued.

Afterwards, I worried about him. He had gone before I finished talking and signing with some other people nearer the front of the shop. I hoped he had not worried about what he said aloud or that he had not been disturbed by the hug. Later that evening, I found out that all was fine, I had merely talked for so long he had had to dart off.

In that moment and afterwards, all of us in the shop had shared a confident vulnerability between ourselves, though I didn't know that was what it was at the time. Confident vulnerability is what I see when people come up to me after shows and offer me their most personal stories. In the past, I would have a burst of confident vulnerability but soon the goblins of regret and anxiety would populate my head.

When I told Jamie about the gig in the bookshop, he said:

'It's connections... it can seem surreal... all these things around us vibrating in wibbly wobbly ways in order to transfer electrical signals from my brain to your brain. We have conversations, we talk, it causes emotions in others, we experience emotions too. And then to be able to recognize that and go give someone the hug they need, or be there for someone.'

All these possibilities. So many missed. So many avoided. So much of our existence can be limited by our vulnerability, but here you are saying, this is what I am and who I am.

There are many people in power looking to exploit your 'weakness'. As we know, weakness is very subjective. If you are open and honest while being able to show that your vulnerabilities may also have strengths, they are robbed of a weapon. In politics, we see potentially good people staying silent when they know they should speak because advisers have told them this will make them vulnerable to the media or their opposition. It is almost impossible to speak genuinely in a world poisoned by relentless bad faith arguments.

As Jamie told me, 'people actually find that they're far more comfortable with a more broken human who's hiding everything than the more exposed honest and happier human'. Many of us are tiptoeing around and getting nowhere but staying blandly safe and unfulfilled.

Jamie sees gaining confident vulnerability as a way of removing an opportunity for people to control or attack you. People do not show their vulnerability because they think they will be handing a weapon to their enemies. When somebody is confident and open with their vulnerability, it makes it far harder to throw their vulnerability back at them.

'You know what you are . . . !'

'Yes, I do.'

'Oh shit.'

Just because you need something does not make you *needy*. In fact, many of the most *needy* people are the very people who spend all their time moaning about the requirements of other people. They are *needy* because they *need* everything to stay the same. What they need all the time is not to be put out in any way, to not have to shift their position in the slightest. Such people place their bags on the seat next to them on a packed train and see anyone asking for them to shift their bag as being the problem as opposed to it being their own selfishness and unsettling attachment to their luggage.

As the neurodivergent movement has become increasingly more visible, many people feel less isolated. As such it gets harder for others to oppress people by saying, 'No one else thinks like this. It's just you who's a freak, and we don't want to make the world better if it is *only* for you.'

As the understanding of autism has broadened and more activists have increased awareness and smashed stereotypes, the stigma of being on the autistic spectrum is being relentlessly challenged. Many of those I have spoken to, who have been diagnosed in middle age, talk of the avoidance of diagnosis when they were young because their parents saw it as the end of their potential. They would be put in a corner and presumed to be of no use. This was all about vulnerability.

Jamie believes that parents of autistic children who discover years later that they're autistic themselves were often more keen to keep hidden the autistic behaviours of their own children because they saw the potential harm and recalled their own necessity to mask and the punishment they received when they didn't. They think they're helping reduce the pain, fearing for their child's vulnerability through their own experience.

Now, more and more people are able to see the power of being vulnerable, confident and safe. The wheelchair user is not the problem when there are only steps into a building – the problem is that no one was thinking about them when they failed to put in a ramp. The person who is disturbed by the lights and noise in a shopping centre is not the problem – the failure to imagine them or their needs is. To be honest, who the hell does like that shopping-centre level of illuminated intrusion? I remember listening to a designer who believed shopping centres were designed to put you on the verge of panic as it would skew your judgement and made you buy rashly.

I spoke to a friend who organizes the National Guardian's Office Freedom to Speak Up Conference which is about 'speaking up about anything that gets in the way of doing a great job'. The organizers always ask delegates about specific requirements they might have and 2024 was the first year where three delegates asked if there could be a quiet room as a place to combat sensory overload. How many people had been attending that conference in the past, knowing they would be vulnerable to sensory overload, but feeling that it was better to say nothing? As more people show their confident vulnerability, so others see that their vulnerability does not make them a pariah. Confident vulnerability says, 'I would like to fit in, but I am not prepared to go through acts of contortion to appear to be what you may expect people to be.'

I believe that my first development of confident vulnerability was not specifically connected to neurodiversity. It was my growing confidence to ask questions of scientists that may have revealed how little I know. So, this is not just about showing your neurodivergent self. I think the world would be better for all of us if we could be our authentic selves. Confident vulnerability should reduce judgement and increase the possibility of progress for all. A world that sees vulnerability as a cudgel to beat people into their place is a mean and lousy world.

Explaining vulnerability to a replicant

Though I sometimes insist that Professor Cox is not a real boy but a *Blade Runner* replicant who would fail the Voight-Kampff test, this is purely for larks and not a true judgement on his character.

In April 2022, I was about to start a tour of North America with Professor Cox. I was going through a lot of anxiety about it. Not the shows, just everything in between. I worried that I would be hit by terrible jet lag and never be able to sleep and so perform terribly. I worried that we had long car journeys and there would be no service stations on the freeway and I would be suffering with food poisoning or some other form of incontinence. I never worried about a plane crash or being shot in the shadowy streets of Chicago, as death is far easier to handle than social shame. I had also just started taking SSRIs (a form of antidepressant) and I had not been warned that, before the foul fog starts to clear, it gets even thicker.

I decided to send the professor an email, not the sort of email that would normally go to a replicant. Much like the email to Josh

MADDER WHEN SANE

about suicidal thoughts, it is something I would never have sent in the past. In the subject line, I called it *Boring email*.

> Hello,
>
> have been debating about sending this email but decided I would and then you can think 'what a nutjob'.
>
> I'm currently experiencing the worst bout of anxiety I've ever had – i think this is because of some rather unhappy news on the family front and just my mind conjuring stuff up.
>
> Find it weird telling you this as you are so much the opposite with your much healthier brain.
>
> sorry, i try to keep this stuff all concealed but I think being honest about it may (or may not) be useful.
>
> Don't worry, on tour I will still be the facile fool I usually am.
>
> See you on Wednesday morning,
>
> Robin

I look at it now and realize that this was actually me on the way out of anxiety, not on the way in. I would never have sent that if I was experiencing my usual energetic anxiety. I would have concealed these feelings. I was confident enough not to hide my fears.

The professor replied.

> Fear not – from the moment we arrive in the fine departure lounge you will be in another world :-)
>
> We'll be boxing in Central Park by the early evening on Wednesday.

Maybe he's a real boy and not a replicant after all.

A few days later, we were in Central Park and we were boxing as quietly as possible. So many people were meditating or doing something mystical with their hands in the air or just humming a Buddhist chant version of something John Lennon said that it felt uncouth to be punching each other too loudly, perhaps leading to collateral misalignment of chakras.

Meds side note

I have not discussed the use of pharmaceuticals in treating neurodivergence. It is a big area, controversial and complicated, and I would rather I was not the one to give you advice, as the complexity of the brain can lead to a complexity of different possibilities in what may or may not be helpful.

Here is my anecdotal experience. About six months after Jamie intervened, I had gained enough confidence to think, 'Why do I allow myself to go through this much anxiety when a daily pill may help?' I was still battling the don't-make-a-fuss-ness of life, but I decided I should give it a go. My doctor prescribed anti-anxiety medication, though I was not warned that the first few weeks may be a little bleaker than usual. However, after four weeks, the differences in my anxiety were tangible.

The reduction in anxiety was eventually vast in pretty much every facet of my life and it remains that way. I have not turned to ADHD meds as I think I have the good fortune to draw on the chaos of my mind for my work. I still toy with the idea and, as a twenty-first-century non-schizoid man, I have taken to the modern potion of mushrooms – in this case lion's mane. I think these shrooms have helped my concentration. It might be psychosomatic, but that's minds for you. There are some days where I feel that a pharmaceutical interruption to my mind's lack of focus may be interesting, but I think I have got to just the right level of conflict and appeasement in my neural pathways for maximum creativity and minimum psychic disturbance.

MADDER WHEN SANE

Back to the story

Many neurodivergent people spend a lot of time thinking about other people's minds because they are trying to work out why other people think what they think and do what they do. I think Philip K. Dick's *Do Androids Dream of Electric Sheep* and the *Blade Runner* films that came from it deal well with the presumption that those that are not human cannot have the same depth of experience. For all their human qualities, replicants are seen as disposable and inferior.

For the autistic community, much was made of their supposed lack of empathy. Donna Williams, who was labelled 'psychotic' when she was two years old, and frequently classed as 'disturbed' throughout her childhood, was an autism advocate who wrote, 'right from the start, from the time someone came up with the word "autism", the condition has been judged from the outside, by its appearances, and not from the inside according to how it is experienced'.[2]

All the pressure and blame of not understanding social interactions and what may appear to be an inability to imagine other people's feelings and the internal experience of others is heaped on the autistic person, but actually, the issue works the other way too. There is the failure of the neurotypical person to be able to imagine the internal experience of the autistic person. The National Autistic Society sums up the problem as 'when people with very different experiences of the world interact with one another, they will struggle to empathize with each other'. When you are no longer masking, that struggle to understand each other can be exacerbated. Many seem to rest easy when they consider autistic people 'not like us', failing to go on the adventure of finding out how they differ and where they are the same.

NORMALLY WEIRD AND WEIRDLY NORMAL

Am I an arsehole?

I am not very adept at being institutionalized, and failing to follow the institution's rules is the kind of thing that can get you incarcerated. I have greater confidence now in expressing opinions about politics and the world around me, which sometimes gets me into trouble with bigger institutions who often like their employees to keep their heads down and their tongues still when anything contentious arises.

Nine months into being much happier, I had lunch with my agent. He likes lunch and so do I, so we get on well. It was a beautiful Italian restaurant and my agent knew the waiter. Oddly, this restaurant was entirely empty except for us. My agent sat down and it was too late for me to take the seat that was looking at the door, as Tony Soprano would have, to make sure that I saw the assassin first, so I ordered my carrot soup and got ready for the hit. The hit turned out to be that two BBC executives had been in contact with my agent to say they believed that I was having some kind of mental health episode and that I should seek help. I was initially floored, then flummoxed, then deeply frustrated and, eventually, as the weeks continued, caught between melancholy and anger. I felt a sense of betrayal but wondered too whether I was entirely innocent. I had argued with my producer on the phone a few days before and been so frustrated that I put the phone down. I began to worry that, without realizing it, I might have been behaving like an arsehole during the making of the shows. Maybe I was a nightmare to work with. Maybe the team had been working with a wild lunatic who only believed he was friendly and courteous.

Later on, I found out about what had provoked this intervention and I realized that it was a case of me getting better on the inside but being presumed to be getting worse by people on the outside. Like *Invasion of the Body Snatchers*, it seemed there was something just not quite right about me. My new confidence when making *The Infinite Monkey Cage* had created worry in the BBC rather than being seen as a positive sign, as if I was going through a disturbing manic phase before the inevitable fall. Their concern helped me realize how we become very used to how someone appears to be, and how unsettling it can be, however positive the change, when they don't seem to be their 'normal' self.

I had also written about suicide ideation on my blog, being honest about myself. People had described it as 'brave' or 'bold' but what they really meant was 'I'd have kept that under my hat if it had been me'. Showbusiness, like any industry with a product, can be very sensitive to how the public perceive its product. What if the product looks like its broken? Will people still buy it? I had tried to be sensitive and careful in my piece on suicide ideation. It was not a cry for help but, I hope, a voice saying, 'just in case you are thinking this too, know that you are not the only one'. What I thought was a carefully written piece about something, which is actually quite common, was seen as a possible indication of my own intention to self-harm.

The necessary camaraderie of minds

What I really learned from this was the importance of comrades in mind, of other neurodivergent people, in particular in times of distress or anxiety.

I was at the Slapstick Festival in Bristol, a happy place to be. I could see that I had bitten my nails to the quick and was now nibbling on the skin that made my thumbs – a dangerous thing to do because, as you know, I already have small thumbs so I should not eat any more of them. If I nibble too much, I will revert to no longer being prehensile and will be made to go sit with the marmosets. I had a message from Heidi, someone who I mainly knew as the bassist in The Fallen Women, an all-female tribute band to the legendary band The Fall. I had once been a guest vocalist with them.

She had moved into a house which the former deceased occupant had left full of books, and she thought that I would enjoy a browse and some biscuits. I am not very good at taking time off, but I knew that Heidi was diagnosed on the autistic spectrum and also ADHD and that she was the right kind of person to spend time with. And she had a dog too.

There is a tremendous calming effect that comes from feeling safe with someone else, especially if there is tea, biscuits, a dog or two, and eventually Prosecco. I think this was the first time that it really came home to me the importance in times of distress of finding other minds operating in a neurodivergent manner. We gabbled on, got excited over weird books and beautiful books, kept apologizing for interrupting each other and then noticed that many of the biscuits had been eaten by the dog. Lucky dog, lucky us. This unrestricted freedom gave me a sense of balance in a turmoil where I was imagining the end of my career.

Perhaps, at the end of it all, Ruby Wax was right about the danger of revealing the life of your mind, choose emphysema over ADHD, choose dysentery over depression. But I believe it is still the right thing to do. The more we speak out with honesty, the more firmly others will believe that they can approach the working environment as their authentic selves. After some bumpy ground, we all came to an understanding and we work together as well as we ever did, if not better.

Happiness – where am I now?

In the summer of 2023, as I repeatedly punched a melon until it exploded, I knew how much better I was. This was the Edinburgh Festival and my show *MELONS!*

It was a joyous and revelatory experience for me. *MELONS!* was a return to a show I had put on nineteen years before, my first Edinburgh solo show. A show which I had considered a failure.

MADDER WHEN SANE

The 2004 show ended with me repeatedly punching a melon with the face of a TV personality who had once wronged me on it, and when the pulp was strewn across me and the stage, I would look at the audience in shock and burst into the soul classic 'Mustang Sally' and . . . BLACKOUT. In the 2023 version, this was how I began the show.

While the show of 2004 was criticized as an ill-thought-out dud, *MELONS!* 2023 had the best reviews of my career, and more importantly, there was a joyous audience reaction too. One of my favourite moments was overhearing a woman in the second row saying 'Are you sure we've come to the right show?' perhaps being surprised by seeing a BBC radio science host dealing with a tropical fruit in such a hostile manner. She was won over when I punched a second melon.

The melon, the blackout and 'Mustang Sally' reprised 2004, but the rest of the show was very different. One of the things that made it so different for me was that I no longer had the perpetual critical voice inside my head that would have started to make me crumble after hearing the first bit of doubt coming from the second row. I also knew what I wanted to do and why I wanted to do it. I wanted to connect, and I could connect honestly now because I also knew who I was. Every night was different, almost every night was without anxiety or doubt. I was sure of myself.

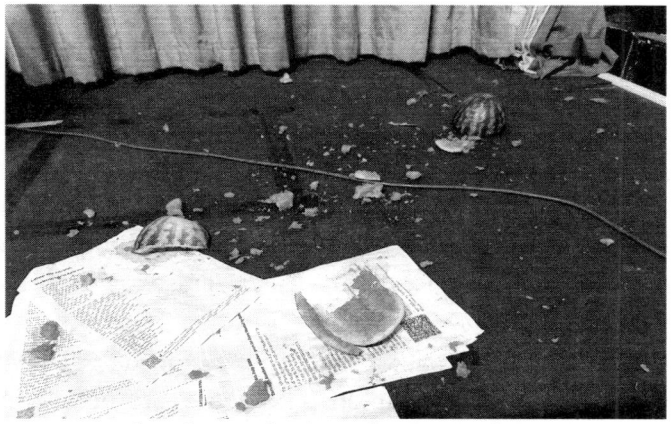

The aftermath of a melon-boxing bout.

NORMALLY WEIRD AND WEIRDLY NORMAL

My performance for many years has been a reflection of the hectic nature of my mind, except with emergency braking whenever the critical voice broke through. Without that voice, I felt I was able to create a truly happy chaos for the first time. The 2004 melon show was also part of what I think is the story of this book. It was doing this failed show that started to make me realize where I had been going wrong. On stage, I had been trying to be what I thought people wanted me to be. As I increasingly became who I was on stage, so began the eighteen-year task of jimmying off the mask in the rest of my life.

These shows felt like the final step to becoming who I could be with my new armament of understanding and the many allies I had found along the way. I was also pleased to win the *Neurodiverse Review*'s ADHD Comedy Award which is hotly contested with so many performers discovering their neurodivergence over the past few years.

I am still getting used to this level of control. To have this grip on so much else allows me to totally let go of the reins when performing – there are no stop signs.

Throwing the coat in the bin

I cannot overstate the transformation in me. There is a moment, sometimes many, every day when I notice a difference in who I am and who I was. When I wake up these days, my first thought is not fear about what I'd done the day before or the dread about the day to come. I no longer have visions of the potential pitfalls ahead of me. When I walk down the street, I don't worry about the judgement of strangers around me.

The past was waking up in that grubby coat, weighing me down with fear, anxiety and sadness, a coat I could never shake off, that influenced all my waking hours, and my dreams and nightmares too. But today, I have woken up and not worried about the day before, something I've said or done, or the stare of another. It makes sense now why people I've met, who have discovered who they truly are and why, always seemed like they were so much lighter and taller. Everything is different.

The most physical feeling of this new lightness came after visiting an exhibition of counter-cultural work at Somerset House in London. It was the confirmation of my new posture. After enjoying the works of Siouxsie Sioux and Derek Jarman, we sat eating carrot cake in the cafe. Suddenly, in an elated, transcendent moment, I was aware of all that I had *not* experienced that morning, all those hourly negative thoughts that had been incessant and insistent for so long. I realized that, when I woke up, my first thought was not about fear of what I'd done the day before to displease someone or the dread of the day to come. I did not see visions of the potential pitfalls ahead.

When I walked down the street, I hadn't worried about the judgement of strangers around me. When I got on the train, I hadn't felt that I must be near the toilet to check it was not out of order just in case I was suddenly startled by a need to go. And when I got into London, I hadn't gone into the station toilets before going on the Tube for similar reasons.* Also, I did not immediately presume that anyone laughing in a group on the carriage was surreptitiously laughing at me.

I walked confidently and happily through the streets, except when a group of slow walkers in front of me expanded to cover the whole pavement, then I was a little grumpy, but I soon told myself to lighten up. My eyes were constantly catching sight of interesting things, a bold and ornate door and a daisy growing through a crack in the pavement that had somehow survived multiple rush hours. When I jovially bought the tickets for the exhibition, I didn't worry

---

* My wife and son both used to find this peculiarity of paranoia very funny. 'He's going to go to the toilet AGAIN!'

that the person behind the counter had made a hasty judgement about what a dick I was.

I was unafraid to occasionally turn to someone who was staring at the same image on a wall as me and make a comment on what I saw. I was not terrified of these shared moments with a stranger. These moments of connection that so many of us want to have but our fear of judgement mutes us. Buying some eccentric books in the gift shop, the assistant and I had a conversation for a few minutes about the work of Louise Bourgeois and the music of The Slits and my mind had no time or space to criticize me, either during the conversation or after. I am even so arrogant as to imagine that we both enjoyed our conversation.

I don't often share too much of my inner life with my wife. She has presumed I am a crackpot for many years now and I would rather be worrying about her than her worrying about me. But today, I could not keep it in and I shared my feeling of elation. She was glad about that and also pointed out that I had some carrot icing on my nose. It was true – I did. It was delicious.

A few weeks later, I was on a train to Sheffield and again was able to connect without fear. As we approached the station, I saw a young woman struggling to get her suitcase off the luggage rack. My first impulse was to help, but immediately, the possible negative interpretations of offering help came into my mind. Would I look patronizing or sexist? Would I look like I was trying to flirt by showing how STRONG I was with my ability to help with luggage? But then my new, better mind popped straight in and said, 'Oh just shut up and help!'

And I did, and she was glad of the help and then she asked me about the badges I was wearing and we talked about art and flowers and Grimsby as the train reached platform 4, and when we said goodbye, I was not worrying about how she may have misinterpreted me. It was a happy and brief connection, a sign that perhaps I am even less anxious now than your average Joe. It feels as if I have used up so much anxiety in my first five decades that now my mind is saying, 'What a relief! That really was getting exhausting. I don't think we'll need to go there again.'

I do sometimes worry there will be an end to this, but there has been a reasonable consistency to this feeling of joy and excitement for three years. Every day, I maintain my awareness of what is different now, what is better now. I think the coat of my past also came with a hessian sack to put over my head that limited the light, because everywhere I walk, I see so much. I am inundated with sensory experiences and excitement.

I know I have been lucky, and that not everyone is transformed by the knowledge and understanding of who they are, for all sorts of different reasons. But I have been told so many beautiful stories of freedom from many who are now on the other side of understanding, whether dyslexia, ADHD, autism or many forms of depression and other mental battles.

Anita told me, 'I let myself experience joy in things, without worrying what others think – I smile and spend time doing things that bring me pleasure and I have almost got rid of the guilt I used to feel when "indulging" my joy.' Her experience is a good example that summarizes many.

Others describe a palpable lightness. Perhaps most importantly, some have expressed a sense of peace. My head hasn't got quieter, but it is now a trampoline rather than a torture chamber.

AFTERWORD

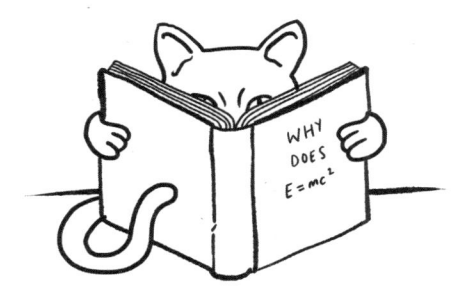

I finished this book while attending Abertoir: The International Horror Festival of Wales. I added my final adjective and then celebrated by attending a screening of *Zombi* with live accompaniment by the composer Fabio Frizzi. Love flowed in between the dismemberments and eye-gouging. The union of the frequently neurodivergent horror fans seemed even more empowering than usual, as the festival was one week after Trump's second presidential victory. The absurdity of zombies was not as absurd as the world itself.

I know that many people, including possibly you, have been hit hard by what appears to be a rubber stamp for regression, for a dismissal of anyone who is seen not to be 'normal enough'.

Even though 'weird' was used by the Democrat campaign to try to insult the Republicans, we know that those who the mainstream most often smears as 'weird' will suffer more under the new administration. Across issues of ethnicity, gender and neurodivergence, existential despair has been evident.

I write this just to remind you that there are many allies ready to support and fight for you and those you love. And for all those who like to sneer at anything deemed as 'woke', keep the actor Kathy Burke's words in mind: 'They're calling you "woke" if you call out bad things, basically. If you're not racist, you're woke. If you're not homophobic, oh, you're woke. Be woke, kids. Be woke. Be wide awake and fucking call it out.'

Or, as she put even more succinctly: 'I love being woke, it's much better than being an ignorant fucking twat.'

Know that there are many people in the world who want more light, more acceptance, more joy and more inclusion for everyone.

While writing this book, I gained a new habit. I have been energetically writing poetry.

It is a good hobby for ADHD people. You see something exciting, your mind fizzes, words pour out, there is just time to finish the poem before your mind gets distracted by a new fascination. One morning, returning from a trip to Slovakia, I was having a hasty back-and-forth of direct messages with the librarian and author Stuart Hennigan. He mentioned the 'dark angels' that haunt so many of us.

This was my reaction.

> *Finally*
> *I clipped the wings of the dark angels*
> *That had fluttered for so long like moths*
> *In the last lone light of night*
> *Once it was black*
> *They were there.*
> *Invisible*
> *But ever-present*
> *They'd beat their wings against the cooling bulb.*
> *Only I could hear the flapping,*
> *But I'd deny there was a sound*
> *For fear of showing weakness.*

AFTERWORD

Then, one day
Now in middle age
I found the way
To quieten down their relentlessness.
I exposed them
By speaking up aloud.
Uncowed.
Not unafraid
But less afraid.
Not bold
But bolder.

Speaking out
They tumbled and twirled like maple seeds
Spinning to the woodland floor.
Not banished
Or vanished.
But unfed
Underfoot
And famished.
So nearly vanquished.
They might still flutter at my heels,
But they can't carry me away
Not now.

To all of you, however your minds may fizz and bubble, I wish you a life unmasked, full of kindness, curiosity and adventure. Let us fight the dark angels together.

ACKNOWLEDGEMENTS

Firstly, I want to thank everyone who was willing to talk to me for this book. There were so many, and I must apologize for not naming you all. Though many of the conversations do not appear in this book, so many are still in my mind, and they continue to build me and change me. Your honesty and willingness to talk was magnanimous.

Thank you to my oldest friends, Joanna Neary, Carl Cooper, Josie Long, Katherine Parker, Carolyn Wilson, Jo Turbitt, Lyndsay Fenner and Trent and Melinda Burton.

Thank you to the authors whose work kept me company, in particular Alexis Pauline Gumbs, Camilla Grudova and Lucia Osborne Crowley.

To Josh Coen, Catherine Loveday, Claudia Hammond, John Higgs and all those who have kept me interested in understanding minds. To Richard Thomas for the wonderful Laugharne festival, and Jeff for being the greatest bookseller.

To Tom Baker, for being the best Doctor and for being a hand up during the down times of school days.

To the musicians who soundtracked my writing, including English Teacher, SPRINTS, This Is the Kit, Cyndi Lauper, John Carpenter, Grace Petrie, Haiku Salut, Tindersticks . . .

Thank you to Charlie Hussey for all the lifts to gigs. To the *Monkey Cage* team. Thank you to Mike, for being foolish enough to edit my book AGAIN.

Thank you to my sisters.

Thank you to my son Archie, always such excellent company, an inspiration and an all-round lovely human.

To Nicki, for working so hard all of the time and for her love.

ENDNOTES

INTRODUCTION

1. Harris, John, 'The mother of neurodiversity: how Judy Singer changed the world', *The Guardian* (2023). https://www.theguardian.com/world/2023/jul/05/the-mother-of-neurodiversity-how-judy-singer-changed-the-world
2. Hendrickx, Sarah, *Women and Girls with Spectrum Disorder* (Jessica Kingsley Publishers, 2015)
3. Baron-Cohen, Simon; Knickmeyer, Rebecca C. and Belmonte, Matthew K., 'Sex differences in the brain: implications for explaining autism', *Science* 310(5749), 819–23 (2005). https://pubmed.ncbi.nlm.nih.gov/16272115/
4. Wells, Angela, *Rash Intruder* (Mills & Boon, 1990)
5. Loehr, Kirsty, *A Short History of Queer Women* (Oneworld Publications, 2022)

CHAPTER 1

1. Davies, Dave, 'Is Your Child an Orchid or a Dandelion? Unlocking the Science of Sensitive Kids', *NPR* (2019). https://www.npr.org/sections/health-shots/2019/03/04/699979387/is-your-child-an-orchid-or-a-dandelion-unlocking-the-science-of-sensitive-kids
2. Arnsten, Amy F. T., 'The Emerging Neurobiology of Attention Deficit Hyperactivity Disorder: The Key Role of the Prefrontal Association Cortex', *Journal of Pediatrics* 154(5), I–S43 (2010). https://pmc.ncbi.nlm.nih.gov/articles/PMC2894421/

ENDNOTES

3   Hunter, Scott J. and Sparrow, Elizabeth P., Executive Function and Dysfunction (Cambridge University Press, 2012) CHAPTER 3: The neurobiology of executive functions. https://www.cambridge.org/core/books/abs/executive-function-and-dysfunction/neurobiology-of-executive-functions/DDE2577AA6B6F6B77377B895711CD20F

4   Freidman, Naomi P. and Robbins, Trevor W., 'The role of prefrontal cortex in cognitive control and executive function', *Neuropsychopharmacology* 47, 72–89 (2022). https://www.nature.com/articles/s41386-021-01132-0

5   Rumball, Freya, 'Post-traumatic stress disorder in autistic people', *National Autistic Society* (2022). https://www.autism.org.uk/advice-and-guidance/professional-practice/ptsd-autism

6   Kearney, Breanne E. and Lanius, Ruth A., 'The brain-body disconnect: A somatic sensory basis for trauma-related disorders', *Frontiers in Neuroscience* 16, 1015749 (2022). https://pmc.ncbi.nlm.nih.gov/articles/PMC9720153/

CHAPTER 3

1   Bauminger, Nirit; Solomon, Marjorie; Aviezer, Anat; Heung, Kelly; Gazit, Lilach; Brown, John and Rogers, Sally J., 'Children with autism and their friends: A multidimensional study of friendship in high-functioning autism spectrum disorder', *Journal of Abnormal Child Psychology* 36, 135–50 (2008). https://doi.org/10.1007/s10802-007-9156-x

2   Petrina, Neysa; Carter, Mark and Stephenson, Jennifer, 'Recent Developments in Understanding Friendship of Children and Adolescents with Autism Spectrum Disorders', in Volkmar, Fred R. (ed.) *Encyclopedia of Autism Spectrum Disorders*, Springer (2021). https://doi.org/10.1007/978-3-319-91280-6_102405

3   Sosnowy, Collette; Silverman, Chloe; Shattuck, Paul and Garfield, Tamara, 'Setbacks and Successes: How Young Adults on the Autism Spectrum Seek Friendship', *Autism in Adulthood* 1(1), 44–51 (2019). https://pmc.ncbi.nlm.nih.gov/articles/PMC8992803/

4   Heidel, Jaime A., 'When a Cactus Meets a Rose – Why Autistic/Neurotypical Friendships Often Fail (And How to Prevent It)', *The*

ENDNOTES

Articulate Autistic (2021). https://www.thearticulateautistic.com/when-a-cactus-meets-a-rose-why-autistic-neurotypical-friendships-often-fail-and-how-to-prevent-it/

CHAPTER 4

1. Mowlem, Florence D.; Skirrow, Caroline; Reid, Peter; Maltezos, Stefanos; Nijjar, Simrit K.; Merwood, Andrew; Barker, Edward; Cooper, Ruth; Kuntsi, Jonna and Asherson, Philip, 'Validation of the Mind Excessively Wandering Scale and the Relationship of Mind Wandering to Impairment in Adult ADHD', *Journal of Attention Disorders* 23(6), 624–34 (2016). https://www.ncbi.nlm.nih.gov/pmc/articles/PMC6429624/

CHAPTER 5

1. Bernstein, Ethan and Waber, Ben, 'The Truth About Open Offices', *Harvard Business Review* (2019). https://hbr.org/2019/11/the-truth-about-open-offices
2. Miserandino, Christine, 'The Spoon Theory', www.butyoudontlooksick.com (2003). https://cdn.totalcomputersusa.com/butyoudontlooksick.com/uploads/2010/02/BYDLS-TheSpoonTheory.pdf
3. Bloom, Nicholas; Liang, James; Roberts, John and Zhichun, Jenny Ying, 'Does Working From Home Work? Evidence from a Chinese Experiment', *National Bureau of Economic Research* 18871 (2013). https://www.nber.org/papers/w18871
4. Brem, Silvia; Grünblatt, Edna; Drechsler, Renate; Riederer, Peter and Walitza, Susanne, 'The neurobiological link between OCD and ADHD', *ADHD Attention Deficit and Hyperactivity Disorders* 6, 175–202 (2014). https://link.springer.com/article/10.1007/s12402-014-0146-x
5. Department for Work and Pensions, 'The Buckland Review of Autism Employment: Report and Recommendations', *Gov.UK* (2023). https://www.gov.uk/government/publications/the-buckland-review-of-autism-employment-report-and-recommendations

ENDNOTES

6   Munanza, Rafiq and Fox, Nikki, 'Autistic People held back by job interview questions – report', *BBC News* (2019). https://www.bbc.co.uk/news/uk-68381352

CHAPTER 6

1   Taylor, Astra (dir.), *Examined Life* (2008)
2   Richardson, Thomas; Jansen, Megan and Fitch, Chris, 'Financial difficulties in bipolar disorder part 2: psychological correlates and a proposed psychological model', *Journal of Mental Health*, 30(1), 3–11 (2019). https://doi.org/10.1080/09638237.2019.1581350
3   Melton, Roy, 'Compulsive spending and bipolar disorder are linked, new Solent NHS Trust study finds', *The News* (2019). https://www.portsmouth.co.uk/health/compulsive-spending-and-bipolar-disorder-are-linked-new-solent-nhs-trust-study-finds-1312788
4   Jones, Rupert, '"Shopping is a nightmare": how ADHD affects people's spending habits', *The Guardian* (2022). https://www.theguardian.com/money/2022/jun/25/shopping-adhd-spending-habits
5   Morley, Carol, 'The amazing undiscovered life of Audrey the artist', *The Guardian* (2016). https://www.theguardian.com/artanddesign/2016/nov/20/carol-morley-discovers-amazing-life-of-artist-audrey-amiss
6   'Hoarding Disorder', *NHS* (2022). https://www.nhs.uk/mental-health/conditions/hoarding-disorder/
7   Yourgrau, Barry, 'Clutter vs. Hoarding vs. Collecting', *Psychology Today* (2015). https://www.psychologytoday.com/gb/blog/mess/201509/clutter-vs-hoarding-vs-collecting
8   'Obsessions and Repetitive Behaviour', *National Autistic Society* (2020). https://www.autism.org.uk/advice-and-guidance/topics/behaviour/obsessions/all-audiences
9   Peak, Eliza, 'The positive impacts playing Dungeons and Dragons has on Mental Health, particularly for people who are Autistic', *Your Voice Heart* (2023). https://yourvoiceheardqyp.wordpress.com/2023/09/16/the-positive-impacts-playing-dungeons-and-

ENDNOTES

dragons-has-on-mental-health-particularly-for-people-who-are-autistic/
10 Leach, Meg, 'How autism powers my D&D', *Polygon* (2021). https://www.polygon.com/22527706/dungeons-dragons-autistic-autism-dungeon-master-essay
11 Manning, Leslie, 'Negotiating *Doctor Who*: Neurodiversity and Fandom', *Media, Margins and Popular Culture* (Palgrave Macmillan, 2015).

CHAPTER 7

1 'The Fairness Imperative – ADHD and Justice Sensitivity', *Edge Foundation*. https://edgefoundation.org/the-fairness-imperative-adhd-and-justice-sensitivity/
2 Caldwell, Marcy, 'Why Am I So Sensitive? Why ADHD Brains Can't Just Ignore Unfairness', *ADDitude* (2022). https://www.additudemag.com/why-am-i-so-sensitive-adhd-in-adults/
3 Schäfer, Thomas and Kraneburg, Thomas, 'The Kind Nature Behind the Unsocial Semblance: ADHD and Justice Sensitivity – A Pilot Study', *Journal of Attention Disorders* 19(8), 715–27 (2012). https://pubmed.ncbi.nlm.nih.gov/23223013/
4 Enright, Jillian, 'Neurodivergents: Justice Warriors', *Invisible Illness* (2021). https://medium.com/invisible-illness/adhders-justice-warriors-9cd2e20eca18
5 Atherton, Gray and Cross, Liam, 'Seeing More Than Human: Autism and Anthropomorphic Theory of Mind', *Frontiers in Psychology* 17(9), 528 (2018). https://www.ncbi.nlm.nih.gov/pmc/articles/PMC5932358/
6 Boren, Ryan, 'Justice Sensitivity', *Stimpunks* (2022). https://stimpunks.org/glossary/justice-sensitivity/
7 Russell, Lucy, 'Black & White Thinking in Autistic Children: Practical Strategies for Parents', *TATF*. https://www.theyarethefuture.co.uk/autism-black-white-thinking/
8 Hattenstone, Simon, 'The transformation of Greta Thunberg', *The Guardian* (2021). https://www.theguardian.com/environment/ng-interactive/2021/sep/25/greta-thunberg-i-really-see-the-

ENDNOTES

value-of-friendship-apart-from-the-climate-almost-nothing-else-matters

9   Solnit, Rebecca, 'Greta Thunberg ends year with one of the greatest tweets in history', *The Guardian* (2022). https://www.theguardian.com/commentisfree/2022/dec/31/greta-thunberg-andrew-tate-tweet
10 Gorowski, Emma, 'Our Autistic Sense of Justice Doesn't Make Us Good People', *Neurodivergent* (2023). https://medium.com/sticks-stones-and-adhd/our-autistic-sense-of-justice-doesnt-make-us-good-people-1463a309d21b

CHAPTER 8

1   Gillette, Hope, 'How Does Autism Affect Sex and Intimacy', *PsychCentral* (2022). https://psychcentral.com/autism/autism-and-sex#autism-and-sex
2   https://www.psychologytoday.com/us/basics/sensory-processing-disorder
3   Needle, Rachel, 'Navigating Neurodiverse Relationships', *Psychology Today* (2023). https://www.psychologytoday.com/gb/blog/mental-and-sexual-health/202308/navigating-neurodiverse-relationships
4   O'Sullivan, Sadhbh, 'I'm Autistic Which Makes Dating Impossible For Me', *Refinery29* (2022), https://www.refinery29.com/en-gb/dating-when-autistic-single-woman
5   patrickmagpie, 'How Do You Ask Your Crush Out?', *NeuroClastic* (2019). https://neuroclastic.com/dating-while-autistic/
6   Hill, Amelia, '"I can only love 100% or 0%": Chris Packham on navigating a neurodiverse relationship', *The Guardian* (2024). https://www.theguardian.com/society/article/2024/jun/03/i-can-only-love-100-or-0-chris-packham-on-navigating-a-neurodiverse-relationship#img-1
7   Headley Ward, John and Curran, Sarah, 'Self-harm as the first presentation of attention deficit hyperactivity attention disorder in adolescents', *Child and Adolescent Mental Health* 26(4), 303–9 (2021). https://acamh.onlinelibrary.wiley.com/doi/full/10.1111/camh.12471

ENDNOTES

8 Eyre, Olga; Langley, Kate; Stringaris, Argyris; Leibenluft, Ellen; Collishaw, Stephan and Thapar, Anita, 'Irritability in ADHD: Associations with depression liability', *Journal of Affective Disorders* 215, 281–7 (2017). https://www.ncbi.nlm.nih.gov/pmc/articles/PMC5409953/

9 Hayden, Chloé, *Different, Not Less: A neurodivergent's guide to embracing your true self and finding your happily ever after* (Murdoch Books, 2023)

10 Klonsky, E. David; Dixon-Luinenburg, Titania and May, Alexis M., 'The critical distinction between suicidal ideation and suicide attempts', *World Psychiatry* 20(3), 439–41 (2021). https://www.ncbi.nlm.nih.gov/pmc/articles/PMC8429339/

11 Van Eck, Kathryn; Ballard, Elizabeth; Hart, Shelley; Newcomer, Ali; Musci, Rashelle and Flory, Kate, 'ADHD and Suicidal Ideation: The Roles of Emotion Regulation and Depressive Symptoms Among College Students', *Journal of Attention Disorders* 19(8), 703–14 (2014). https://journals.sagepub.com/doi/abs/10.1177/1087054713518238

12 Kakuszi, Brigitta; Bitter, István and Czobor, Pál, 'Suicidal ideation in adult ADHD: Gender difference with a specific psychopathological profile', *Comprehensive Psychiatry* 85, 23–9 (2018). https://www.sciencedirect.com/science/article/abs/pii/S0010440X18300968

13 Cassidy, Sarah; Bradley, Paul; Robinson, Janine; Allison, Carrie; McHugh, Meghan and Baron-Cohen, Simon, 'Suicidal ideation and suicide plans or attempts in adults with Asperger's syndrome attending a specialist diagnostic clinic: a clinical cohort study', *The Lancet Psychiatry* 1(2), 142–7 (2014). https://www.thelancet.com/journals/lanpsy/article/PIIS2215-0366(14)70248-2/fulltext

CHAPTER 9

1 Johnson, Joe; Morris, Sarah and George, Sanju, 'Misdiagnosis and missed diagnosis of adult attention-deficit hyperactivity disorder', *BJPsych Advances*, 27(1), 60–1 (2020). https://www.cambridge.org/core/journals/bjpsych-advances/article/misdiagnosis-and-

ENDNOTES

missed-diagnosis-of-adult-attentiondeficit-hyperactivity-disorder/FF6646643B2BC02FFE7D20BBB4967950
2. https://www.quora.com/Does-unstable-self-image-have-something-to-do-with-autism

CHAPTER 11
1. Weisz Carrington, Gabriel, *The Invisible Painting: My Memoir of Leonora Carrington* (Manchester University Press, 2021)

CHAPTER 12
1. Kellaway, Kate, 'Ruby Wax: "I've spent a lifetime giving the illusion all is well. It wasn't and it isn't"', *The Guardian* (2023). https://www.theguardian.com/tv-and-radio/2023/may/07/ruby-wax-not-as-well-as-i-thought-i-was-depression-interview-cast-away
2. Williams, Donna, *Autism: An Inside-Out Approach* (Jessica Kingsley Publishers, 1996)

INDEX

Page numbers in **bold** refer to illustrations;
page numbers in *italics* refer to footnotes.

65daysofstatic 73

Abertoir: The International
    Horror Festival of Wales 150,
    247
Aberystwyth 150
abseiling 35
abuse
    abusive relationships 15–16,
        160–1, 170, 221
    childhood 33–4, 47
    parental 33–4, 74
    physical 39, 47, 74
    psychological 47
    sexual 39
accents 55
activism 159–60
Adam Ant 171
ADD *see* attention deficit disorder
addiction 33–4, 223
ADHD *see* attention deficit
    hyperactivity disorder

administration 124
agency 28
agoraphobia 214
alcohol consumption 100
Alexandra 104
alexithymia 219, *219*
Alice 125
alienation 52, 157–8
Allen, Dave 110–11
alpha pack 55
American Beauty (1999) *192*
Amiss, Audrey 138
amygdala 33, 34–5
Anderson, Lindsay 69
anger issues 34, 47, 66, 178–9,
    184, 220
animals 156–7
Anita 245
Annelies 58, 59
anthropomorphism 156–7
anti-anxiety medication 184, 236
anti-bullying organizations 54

259

INDEX

antidepressants 234
anxiety 32, 116, 118, 203, 215, 217–18
 and anger 178
 attitudes towards 214
 and childhood trauma 47
 and compulsive spending 135
 'cure' for 18, *18*
 and dating 170
 financial 136
 and hoarding 139
 and inner dialogue 12
 and irritability 179
 and manipulation 16, 163
 and masking 7, 9–10
 maternal 31, 45
 medication for 236
 and neurodivergent diagnosis 12, 212, 220, 225
 performance 234, 235
 perpetual 118
 and the prefrontal cortex 37
 and realizing other people think that you are weird 72
 regarding the happiness of others 153
 and remuneration 116
 residual 62, 185
 social 81, 111
 and social rules 7
 and support 239
 and therapy 187–8, 189–90, 193, 197
 and the transformations of diagnosis 242–3, 245
 and trauma 26, 28
 and vulnerability 230
apologies 162
ASD *see* autism spectrum disorder
Asperger's syndrome
 and depression 183
 diagnosis 224
 and suicidal ideation 183
 see also autism spectrum disorder
'Aspie supremacy' 160
Astaire, Fred 16
Atherton and Cross 156–7
attention
 dysregulation 123, 127
 paying 59–61
 see also inattention
attention deficit disorder (ADD) 143, 178
 see also attention deficit hyperactivity disorder
attention deficit hyperactivity disorder (ADHD) 6, 8, 21–2, 40, 202, 245, 248
 ADHD, hyperactive 194
 ADHD, inattentive 154, 194
 and alcohol use 100
 and anger 178
 and boredom 123
 chaos of 130–1, 196
 as childhood disorder 194
 comorbid with ASD 22, 55, 86–7, 108, 123, 127, 221–2, 240
 comorbid with autism 86–7, 180
 comorbid with OCD 123, 140

INDEX

and conversation 94–5, 96–9
cynical attitudes towards 212
and deadlines 105–6
and depression 182
diagnosis 11–13, 19, 56, 120, 127, 201–9, 211, 213–15, 218–25
dismissive attitudes towards 212
and Edinburgh Fringe 242
and emotion 37, 46, 119
and executive function 37
and form-filling 124
and intensity of feeling 159
and justice sensitivity 153–5
medication 108, 184, 212, 236
misdiagnosis 73, 194
and negative messages 161
and object permanence 86–7
and obsessions 143
and ordering information 37
over-diagnosis 19
and overspending 135, 136
and passion 97–8
racing thoughts of 93, 94, 100–1, 127, 205
and rejection 81
and relationships 86–7, 167, 169
and self-harm 175
and a sense of jeopardy 105
and a sense of self 195–6
and sitting still 56
and suicidal ideation 182–3, *182*
and trauma 34
undiagnosed 74, 194
and the workplace 108, 112–13, 123–5
see also attention deficit disorder
attention tunnels 108, 110
Atwood, Margaret 6
authors/authorship 123, 126–7, 174–5, 248–9
autism 4, 8, 10, 13, 73, 75, 195, 201–3, 245
and activism 159–60
and anthropomorphism 156–7
and burnout 109
comorbid 39, 86–7, 123, 140, 180
and conversation 97–8
diagnosis 14, 212, 213, 218–24, 227
and eye contact 58
fatigue of 109
and form-filling 124
and justice sensitivity 160
as 'male' condition 14, 219
masking 14
and obsessions/passions 98, 143, 148
and perfectionism 122
and PTSD 39
and rejection 81
and relationships 84, 86–7
and role-playing games 147
and romantic relationships 167, 169, 170–1
and self-blame 160–1
and self-knowledge 185

INDEX

autism (cont'd)
  and social outsiders 145
  stereotypes of 2, 158, 232–3
  and stigma 232–3
  and suicide 183
  undiagnosed 74
  and the workplace 108–11, 113, 122, 124
  see also autism spectrum disorder
autism spectrum disorder (ASD) 8, 14
  comorbid with ADHD 22, 55, 86–7, 108, 123, 127, 221–2, 240
  and conversation 96–7
  diagnosis 219, 220, 221, 222–4
  and emotional regulation 46
  and exams 61
  and eye contact 58
  and fidgeting 56–7
  and friendship 83–4
  and intensity of feeling 158–9
  misdiagnosis 73
  and romantic relationships 169, 170–2
  and suicidal ideation 183
  and theory of mind 156–7
  tidiness of 130
  and trauma 39
  and the workplace 125
  see also Asperger's syndrome; autism
Autistica 124
autonomy, workplace 115–16
autopilot 109, 196

Baldwin, James 157
banter 68, 85, 162
Bauminger, Solomon, Aviezer, Heung, Gazit et al. 83
BBC 157, 238–9, 241
  science unit 105
Beckett, Samuel 182, 186
Becky 122
Belper 6
bereavement 26–7, 31, 34, 176
Beth 101, 122–3
Beverly Hills 90210 (TV show) 186
Bible 46
biodiversity 8
bipolar disorder 13, 135–6, 209, 209, 225
  comorbid 22, 135, 138
  see also manic depression
Blade Runner films 234, 237
Blake, William 23
Blower, Lisa 118
Bob 123
body language 169
boredom 10, 62, 63, 123, 137, 140
Borissova, Anya 51
Bosch, Hieronymus, *Garden of Earthly Delights* 98
bottling up 98–101
Bourgeois, Louise 244
Boyce, W. Thomas 35
Brahe, Tycho *190*
brain 34
  and the battle for focus 91–4
  complexity 26

INDEX

downstairs (subconscious) 32, 33
injury 46
and justice sensitivity 154
racing 91–4
and relationships 80–1
and risk-taking 34–5
upstairs (conscious) 32, 33
see also amygdala; frontal lobe
brain lesions 30, 31
brain tumour 322
brainstem 47
Breakfast Club, The (1985) 144–5
Bremner, Rory 208
Bride of Frankenstein (1935) 150
'brokenness' 197, 213, 218, 221–3, 232, 239
Brontë, Emily 6
Buckland Review of Autism and Employment, The 124
Buddha 21
Buddhism 21
bullying 15, 35, 39, 54, 63–4, 66–71, 74, 75, 85, 155, *155*, 221
  instigated by teachers 60–1, 72
Buñuel, Luis 27
Burke, Kathy 247–8
burnout 109
Burton, Trent 176–7
Butler, Samuel 46

Cade 221–2
Cage, John 21
Caldwell, Marcy 154
capitalism 136

carers, young 214
Carpenter, John 100
Carrington, Gabriel Weisz 212–13
Carrington, Leonora 213
Centers for Disease Control and Prevention 182
cerebral palsy 3
change
  fear of 213
  resistance to 19
chaos 28, 106, 130–3, **132**, 138–42, 150, 173, 175, 178, 185, 196–7, 199, 207–8, 227, 236
'character-building' 70
Charlie (author's school friend) 66, 70–1
Charlotte 151–2
Chatterton, Thomas 184
Chelmsford 38
Cheltenham College 69
childhood abuse 33–4, 47
  sexual 33
childhood development 37–8
childhood experience 25, 27–34, 36, 52, 221, 230
  and executive function 37, 39
  and expectations 40
  and shame 48–9
  and somatic sensory processing dysfunction 46–7
  talking through 41–4, 46–7
  and weirdness 66–7
children 219–20, 233
Chris 95

INDEX

chromosomes, Y 8
Clare, Tim 122
Clark, Karen 148
climbing, free climbers 34–5
clubs 74
cluttering 142–3
cocaine 216
cognitive dissonance 21, 66
Coldplay 100
collections 129–44, 180
Columbo 149
comorbidity 22, 39–40, 55, 86–7, 108, 123, 127, 135, 138, 140, 180, 221–2, 240
compassion 70, 201, 230–1
competitiveness 79
comprehension difficulties 96–7
compromise 66–7
compulsions 123, 135–6
confidence illusion 117–19
confident vulnerability 230–4
conformity 57–8, 62, 67, 70, 72, 112
Confucius 32
connection
   experience of a lack of 66
   fear of 244–5
   need for 40, 244–5
   and role-playing games 147
   workplace 104
conscious awareness 47
control issues 15–16, 28, 32, 47, 169, 170, 178
conversations 91–101
   bottling up 98–101
   interrupting 94–5

neurotypical 94
   and passions 97–8
   rules of 87–8, 89
   workplace 104, 105
   see also speech
coping mechanisms 14, 199
Corney, Charlotte 172
COVID pandemic 113, 114, 176–7, 199–204
Cox, Brian 1, 118, 126, 234–6
creativity 21, 23, 96, 118–19, 122–4, 208
   and chaos 142
   and flow states 104
   and letting off steam 101
   women and 5
   and the workplace 108, 126–7
criminality 33–4
Cronenberg, David 96
Cunliffe, Michael 79
Cure, The 177
Curmi, Alex 214–16
Cusack, James 124
Cushing, Peter 27, 45
Cutler, Ivor 80

dad 27, 29, 31, 41–5, **44**, 48–9, 51–2, 134, 136–7, 149, 156–8, 222, 230
'dandelion' metaphor 34–6
Danielle 145–6
dating 165–6, 169–71
Davies, Russell T. 148
Davis, Sammy, Jr 127
deadlines 105–6, 122
deception 2–3

264

INDEX

decluttering 142–4
dementia 50
Democrats 247
Denning, Lord 41
depression 10, 28, 30–1, 118, 153, 190, 217, 245
   and Asperger's syndrome 183
   attitudes towards 214
   comorbid 183, 221
   diagnosis 223
   maternal 31, 45, 50
   and suicide 182
   and therapy 187–8
'depression liability' 179
Derbyshire, Delia 148
despair 19, 26, 36, 39, 50, 63, 119, 153, 176, 184, 247
diagnosis 11–13, 40, 211–27
   ADHD 11–13, 19, 56, 120, 127, 201–9, 208, 211, 213–15, 218–25
   ASD 219, 220, 221, 222–4
   depression 223
   disclosure 208–9, 240
   late 86, 95, 97, 123, 160, 212–13, 229, 233
   and masking 208–9
   negative experiences of 219–21
   relief of 224–5
   resentment towards 220
   revelation of 201–9
   transformations of 226–7, 242–5
Dick, Philip K. 195, 237
Diesel, Vin 92
difference, threat of 75

discomfort, of other people 154–5
dishonesty 56, 87–8
distress 239, 240
diversity 7–8
Doctor Who franchise 148–9
Dodson, William 161
doodling 59
Doom bags/boxes 133–4, 136–7
dopamine 154
drug use 100, 216
   and addiction 33–4
Duncan, Michelle 158
Dungeons & Dragons (role-playing game) 146–8
Dunja 74
dyslexia 8, 111, 245
   comorbid 22
   and creativity 126
   diagnosis 213
   and form-filling 124
dyspraxia 8, 111
   comorbid 22
   diagnosis 213, 218, 221–2

eccentricity 20, 32–3, 209, 229–30
Ed (author's school friend) 67–71, 94
Edinburgh 142, 157
Edinburgh Fringe Festival 86, 240–2
educational psychologists 73
Einstein, Albert 23
Elephant Man, The (1980) 52

INDEX

Elizabeth II 138
Elizabeth 91
emails 114–15
emotional circuitry 119
emotional impulsivity 154
emotional liability 154
emotions
   and alexithymia 219, *219*
   dysregulation 175–8
   hiding 72
   intensity of 158–9
   negative 40
   processing 37
   regulation 46, 51–2
   sharing 51
   see also specific emotions
empathy 36, 70, 93, 153, 156, 161, 237
emptiness 195
energy levels 10, 72, 95, 107, 109, 112, 118, 159, 176, 178, 196, 209
Enright, Jillian 154
Esme 123
Estevez, Emilio 145
ethics 67
ethnicity 55, 247
   see also race
Evans, Milly 169
Everest, Mount 10
evolutionary theories 5
exams 61
Executive Decision (1996) 37
executive function 36–40, 80–1, 123, 127, 158, 175, 215
expectations 4–5, 40, 54, 84

experience 4–5, 10, 25–6
   see also childhood experience; trauma
eye contact 58, 69, 169

failure
   fear of 213, 223
   feelings of 40, 120–1, 122, 178, 206, 207
   to 'fit in' 7, 15, 62, 153, 163, 209
fairness 67, 153–6, *155*, 158–60, 163, 222
Fall, The 239
Fallen Women, The 239–40
Fast and the Furious, The (2001) 92
fear 2, 11, 26, 28, 34–5, 47, 75, 197, 218, 242–3
   of ADHD 212
   of change 213
   of connection 244–5
   of failure 213, 223
   of judgement 244
   of making people unhappy 40
   of rejection 80–3, 168–9, 223
   spectrum of 34
Ferguson-Walker, Clare 225
Fernyhough, Charles 92–3
fidgeting 56–8
'fight or flight' response 47, 217
finishing, failure to 122
'fitting in' 10
   failure to 7, 15, 62, 153, 163, 209
   see also social outsiders
flirting 169

INDEX

flow states 104, 108, 110, 125
focus 94, 105, 108, 110
   battle for 91–4, 123
   and drug use 216
   intense 125
   lack of 126, 236
form-filling 124
Frankenstein (1910) 150
free climbers 34–5
Free Solo (documentary) 34
Freud, Sigmund 194
friendship 65, 67–71, 77–89, 220
   and banter 162
   definition 83
   expectations of 84
   need for 84, 88–9
   neurodivergent circles 95, 209, 224, 239–40
   neurotypical 224
   overthinking 85–6
   rules of 83–6, 89
   and therapists 186, 196–7
   and the transformations of diagnosis 226–7
'friendship degradation mechanics' 87
Frizzi, Fabio 247
frontal lobe 37

gay men 17–18
   see also LGBT people
Geller, Uri 98–9
gender issues 3, 5, 23, 247
genetics 25
gods 3
Godzilla 130

Gorowski, Emma 160
goths 72, 145–6
grandfather 222
grief 191, 223
Guardian, The (newspaper) 159, 229
guilt 28, 33, 48, 49, 71, 151–3, 161, 218, 245
Guns N' Roses 92

Haig, Matt 224
Hammersmith Apollo 126
Hands of the Ripper (1971) 150
happiness 213–14, 216–17, 232, 240–2
   focus on other people's 40, 153, 167, 189–91, 200
   see also unhappiness
Harris, Joanne 116
Harrison, George 165
Harvard Business Review 104
Haverfordwest Library 109
Hayden, Chloé 75, 180–1
health, spoon theory model of 107–8
Heather 161
Hegel, Georg Wilhelm Friedrich 135
Heidel, Jaime A. 87
Heidi 239–40
Hendrickx, Sarah 14
Hennigan, Stuart 248
hierarchies 50, 56, 79, 103, 104
Himba tribe 5
Hines, Gregory 127
hoarding 130–44, **131**, 180

INDEX

hobbies 137, 143, 248
Holly 74
homelessness 221
honesty 56, 170, 240
horror genre 149–50
House (TV series) 149
human condition, weirdness of 1–2, 23
human rights 8
Hunter, Scott J 37–8
hyperactivity 194
hyperverbosity 162
hypomania 130–1
hysteria 8–9

Idle, Eric 119
If (2024) 69
imposter syndrome 121, 223
inattention 86
Ince, Robin
  ADHD diagnosis 11–12, 201–9, 211
  on being alone as a child 77–80
  and body image 64, *64*
  book tours 109
  childhood car crash 27–31, 36, 39–45, 49–51, 230
  creative pursuits 101, 103
  difficult behaviour 238–9
  dreams 27
  and friendships 65, 67–71, 79, 81, 81–2
  and his mum 26–31, 41–5, 48–9, 50–2, 63, 65, 137, 156, 190, 192, 230
  and his wife 1, 9, 52, 88, 94, 129, 133, 140, 165, 171–2, 175–7, 181, 200, 204, 209, 227, *243*, 244
  live shows 1, 11, 13, 30, 103, 105–6, 117–18, 197, 200, 207–8, 230–1, 234, 235, 239–42, **242**
  love of showing off 20, 28–9, 81, 177, 185
  on material success 115–17
  path to the comedian's stage 30
  post-show accessibility 82, 115
  and romantic relationships 80, 165–6
  and school 60–71, 65, 67–71, 80, 81, 183, 199
  and sport 46, 60, 61, 64, 68, 79
  and therapy 30, 185–97, 199, 203
  and the transformations of diagnosis 242–5
Infinite Monkey Cage, The (radio show) 118, 239
info-dumping 169–70
injustice 55–6, 153–6, 158–9
ink pens, horror of 61
inner voice 23, 121, 206, 216
  critical 12–13, 15, 18, 83, 117–19, 242
  eccentric 20
Inside No. 9 (TV series) 52
Institute for Challenging Disorganization 142

INDEX

institutions 54
   difficulties with 238
interiority (inner life) 2, 4, 20, 23
   abusive 15–16
   see also inner voice
International Space Station 177
intimacy 167, 203
Invasion of the Body Snatchers (1978) 238–9
irritability 179
irritable bowel syndrome (IBS) 193
isolation 232
   see also loneliness

Jamie and Lion *see* Knight, Jamie
Janey (author's eldest sister) 30, 41, 42–3, **43**, 45, 50, 51, 63, 137, 139
Jarman, Derek 243
Jason 98
Jeevi 73
Jesus 155–6
Jo (author's friend) 16–18
Joel (author's friend) 98–9, 101
John Peel Show (radio show) 80
Johnny (author's friend) 150
Jojo 74
Josefina 170
Josh (therapist) 186, 188–9, 190–1, 199–201, 234–5
Josie 155–6, 158
joy 245
judgement 218, 234, 244
Julia 94–5, 104, 105

Jungian truth bowl 192, *192*
justice sensitivity 153–6, *155*, 158–60
Justine (author's friend) 60

Kant, Immanuel, *Critique of Pure Reason* 12
Karen-Ann 100
Kathryn 219, 223–4
Katie 122
Kearney and Lanius 47
Kellogg's Frosties 138
Kelly, Gene 16
Kerns, Connor 39
Kierkegaard, Søren 135
kindness 36, 105, 222, 249
kinetic energy 107
Knight, Jamie (Jamie and Lion) 85, 108, 109–11, 157, 184, 201–9, 211, 214, 216, 217, 230, 231–2, 233, 236
Kondo, Marie 142–3, 144

Lancaster, Sophie 53–4, 75
Lancaster, Sylvia 53–4, 75
Lanchester, Elsa 150
Lansbury, Angela 113
Latitude Festival 118
laws 3
Leach, Meg 147
Leah 146
Lee, Christopher 45
Lennon, John 236
leprosy (Hansen's disease) 188, *188*
lesbians 17–18, 157

INDEX

LGBT people 10, 148, 157, 166
  see also gay men; same-sex relationships; trans people
Lighthouse Bookshop, Edinburgh 157
Limburg, Joanne 140
lion's mane mushrooms 236
Lizzie (author's friend) 72
Loehr, Kirsty, *A Short History of Queer Women* 17–18
Lolo 142
loneliness 62, 65, 74, 153
  see also isolation
loners 77–80, 89, 103, 166
Long, Josie 93
Lord of the Flies, The (Golding) 55
love 165–77
Lowe, Alice 5
Lowestoft 20
lupus 107
Lynch, David 12

Mabel (author's friend) 72, 73
McAnulty, Dara 4
McDonald's 138
McDowell, Malcolm 69
McGoohan, Patrick *149*
McKelvie, Jamie 130
McKenna, Virginia 65
madness 95–7
  quiet 32–3
  see also mental health; *specific conditions*
Magic Eye pictures 206–7, *207*
Mairi 157

Man, Myth and Magic magazine 138, *138*
mania 134–8, 239
  see also hypomania
manic depression 214
  see also bipolar disorder
manipulation 15, 16, 121, 213
marginalization 157–8
Maria 74
Martinez, Francesca, *What the F*** Is Normal?* 3
masking 7, 9–11, 14, 15, 22, 63, 70, 168, 237, 249
  and diagnosis 208–9
  and eye contact 58
  failures 63
  and the risk of other people thinking that you are weird 72
  and romantic relationships 171, 172
  and a sense of self 195–6
  and the transformations of diagnosis 226
  and the workplace 120
Matt 120–1
Matty 143–4
Maudsley, The 214–15
medication 108, 184, 212, 225, 236
meetings 111–13
MELONS! shows 240–2, **242**
meltdowns 38–9, 45–6, 48, 174–81
  see also tantrums
memory, working 37

INDEX

mental health 34
  attitudes towards 214
  battle with 47
  burden of 217–18
  discrimination regarding 229–30
  polarized nature 8
  see also madness; *specific conditions*
messiness 130–3, **132**, 138–42, 175, 196
Middleton, Ellie 127
Mills and Boon 16–17
Milner, Leah 136
Mind Excessively Wandering Scale (MEWS) 99–100
miracles 188
Miserandino, Christine 107–8
misogyny 70
money management issues 135–7
Monk 149
Morley, Carol 138
Morris, Joel 146
Morrison, Toni 6
mothers
  abusive 33–4, 74
  see also mum
Motors, The 37
Mount Florida Books 230
Mr Inbetween (TV show) 52
Mudhoney 100
Mulholland Drive (2001) 12
mum 41–5, **44**, 48–52, **49**, 63, 65, 137, 156
murder 5, 31, 34, 53–4
Murder, She Wrote (TV show) 113

music 100, 146
'Mustang Sally' (song) 241

Namibia 5
narcissism 28, 35, 222
National Autistic Society (NAS) 143, 237
National Guardian's Office Freedom to Speak Up Conference 233
National Health Service (NHS) 138, 183, 187–8
Neary, Joanna 86–7, **86**, 140
Needle, Rachel 167
needy people 232
Neeson, Liam *109*
Neff, Megan Ann 109, 123
negative intent attribution 154
negative messages 161
Neil 125
nematodes 26
neural networks 37
neurodivergence 6, 7–15, 17–18, 22–3, 25, 31, 36, 130–1, 202–3, 205, 237, 247
  and abusive relationships 161
  and apologies 162
  and banter 85
  blindness to 14–15
  and comorbidity 39–40
  and confident vulnerability 232, 234
  and conversation 94–5, 96–7, 97, 101
  and creativity 126

INDEX

neurodivergence (*cont'd*)
    diagnosis 11–13, 20, 207, 209, 211–13, 216–17, 220
    dismissive attitudes towards 229
    energy expenditure of 109, 110
    failure to understand neurotypicals 237
    and goths 145–6
    and guilt 151–2
    and hoarding 139
    and marginalization 7
    and masking 7, 9–11
    and medication 236
    and neurodivergent circles 95, 209, 224, 239–40
    and obsessions 148–9, 150
    other people's stories of 71–5, 82
    and overspending 136
    racing thoughts of 92, 94
    and relationships 77, 81, 85, 87–8
    and role-playing games 146
    and romantic relationships 166–72
    sense of justice and fairness 153–4, 159
    and sensory sensitivity 46
    as taboo 50
    and weirdness 55–6, 58, 69, 71, 73–4
    and work 104, 107–9, 112, 114–18, 120–2, 124, 126, 128
    see also specific types of neurodivergence

Neurodiverse Review 242
neurodiversity movement 8
neuroscience 7, 23
neuroticism 151
neurotypicals, failure to understand neurodivergence 237
Newley, Anthony 182
Nick Cave and the Bad Seeds 145
nicknames 55
Nilsson, Harry 42
Nimoy, Leonard 68
non-binary people 9, 147
non-verbal communication 84–5
    see also body language; eye contact
'normal' 54
    battle to be 208, 209
    changing attitudes towards 6–7
    deviations from 56
    as not necessarily a good thing 71
    as relative term 6–7
    unbearable rules of being 3–7, 8, 20–1
novelty-seeking 123, 139–40
Numan, Gary 66

object permanence 86–7
objects
    attachments to 180–1
    see also hoarding
O'Brien, Edna 6
obsessions 98, 123, 130–1, 134–9, 143–50, 159, 162
obsessive-compulsive disorder (OCD) 214

INDEX

comorbid 123, 140
OCD-like behaviours 32
Octavia (therapist) 55–6, 72–3, 88–9, 223
office politics 104
Ogle, Charles *150*
Ono, Yoko 133
open plan offices 104–5, 114
Orbison, Roy 120
'orchid' metaphor 35–6
order 36, 37, 130–2, 139
organizational skills 37
Osmond, Donnie 48
other people's stories
   about conversation 94–5
   about diagnosis 219–23
   about the neurodivergent experience 71–5, 82
   about workplaces 122–7
overwhelm 85, 230

Packham, Chris 84–5, 172
pain 28, 36
   emotional 9–10, 35, 36, 47, 49, 222, 230
   self-report measure of centralized 46
Paolozzi, Sir Eduardo 142
paperwork 124
parent–child relationship, traditional 50
passion/passions 97–8, 113, 129, 150, 155, 159
Paul (author's friend) 160–1
Peak, Eliza 146–7
peer pressure, resistance to 159

'penguin pebbling' 169
Penthouse magazine 137
people-pleasing 40, 167
perfectionism 14–15, 122
Perry, Philippa 35
Perry, Sarah 38–9
personal space 104–5
Peterson, Jordan B. 140, 144, 155
phobias 214
physical abuse 39, 47, 74
Plato 122, 206
poetry-writing 248–9
Poitier, Sidney 89
politics 104, 151–63, 231–2, 238, 247
popularity 79
post-traumatic stress disorder (PTSD) 25, 26, 39, 46–7
power 163, 169
powerlessness 178
prefrontal cortex ('the personality centre') 37–8, 40, 80–1, 171, 179
Preston, Billy 42
Prevenge (2016) 5, *5*
Price, Christopher 176, *176*
Price, Vincent 133, 205
Priestley, Jason 186
Prisoner, The (TV series) 149, *149*
prisons 54, 60, 221
problem-solving 126
procrastination 61, 125
productivity 113
Proust, Marcel 42
psychological abuse 47

INDEX

psychological labelling 21, 22
psychology 23
PTSD *see* post-traumatic stress disorder

Quavers 138
quiet rooms 233

race 23, 156, *156*, 157, 247
   see also ethnicity
Rash Intruder (Mills and Boon romance) 16
Rauschenberg, Robert 21
Reading 83
real, not feeling 195–6
Reality Tunnel (radio series) 20
reclusion 214
recruitment 124–5
Reed, Lou 93
rejection, fear of 80–3, 168–9, 223
rejection sensitive dysphoria (RSD) 81
relationships
   abusive 15–16, 160–1, 170, 221
   breaking up 170
   controlling 15–16
   neurodivergent circles 95, 209, 224, 239–40
   romantic 86–7, 165–77, 205
   sexual 23, 167–8
   see also friendships
religion 55
repetitive behaviours 140
replicants 234–5, 237
Republicans 247

reputations 54–5
resilience 66–71
respect 158, 205
responsibility, sense of 151–2, 197
Richard, Cliff 42
Richardson, Thomas 135–6
risk-taking 34–5
River 58, 59
Robert 227
Robin 123–4
Robocop films 181
role-playing games 146–8
Rosanda 43
Royal College of Psychiatrists 183
Royal Institution 126
Royal Society for the Prevention of Cruelty to Animals (RSPCA) 156
rules 106, 121
   battle of 209
   of being normal 3–7, 8, 20–1, 71
   conversational 87–8, 89
   of friendship 83–6, 89
   and masking 9
   of role-playing games 148
   unjust 55–6
   and weirdness 54
   workplace 103
Rumball, Freya 39
Russell, Bertrand 78
Russell, Lucy 159
Ruth 94

INDEX

sadness 28, 34, 40, 51–2, 153, 182, 225, 230, 242–3
Saline, Sharon 159
Sam 185
same-sex relationships 3
 see also gay men; LGBT people
Sappho 17
Sarah (author's other sister) 27–8, 30, 41–3, 50, 139
Sarah (cosplaying Mad Hatter) 220
Satan 149, *149*
Scanners (1981) 96
Schäfer and Kraneburg 154
schizophrenia 138
schools 54–8, 60–2, 72–4, 199, 221
 boarding 62–71, 80, 183
 and bullying 155
 dining rooms 60
 and friendship 80
Scientologists 191
Scott, Fran 126
Seagal, Steven 37
secrecy 33
selective serotonin reuptake inhibitors (SSRIs) 234
self
 blindness to 13, 14–15
 lack of a sense of 195–6
 sense of 67
self-acceptance 221
self-blame 28–9, 32, 39, 40, 49, 160–1, 197
self-control 37
self-criticism 215
 see also inner voice, critical
self-esteem, low 16, 81, 116, 135
self-expression 96, 101, 170
self-fulfilling prophecies 194
self-harm 175, 239
self-image, unstable 195
self-knowledge/-understanding 15, 21, 25, 118, 185, 197, 216, 220, 222, 227, 245
self-loathing 12, 15, 48–9, 106, 119, 175, 185, 193
self-reliance 167
self-worth 15, 116, 153, 221
sensitivity 35
sensory overload 104–5, 233
sensory sensitivity 5, 46–7, 167, 180–1
Sequeira, Heather 32–3, 46
Seuss, Dr 199
sexual abuse 39
sexual relationships 23, 167–8
shame 2, 23, 33, 40, 48–50, 52, 63, 98, 162, 192, 218, 221, 230, 234
Sheedy, Ally 145
Sheffield 244
showbusiness 229–30, 239
Sickels, Leslie 167
Sievey, Chris 139
Simone, Nina 165
Simple Minds 144
Singer, Judy 7–8
Sioux, Siouxsie 243
sitting still 56–8
Slade 42, 51
Slapstick Festival, Bristol 239–40
sleep difficulties 99

INDEX

sleep issues 129–30, *130*
Slits, The 244
smartphones 115
Smith, Ali 89
Smith, Robert 177
social anxiety 85, 111
social class 23
social cues, difficulties with 84–5, 121
social exclusion 72
social interaction, lack of understanding regarding 237
social outsiders 7, 15, 62, 144–5, 153, 163, 209
  see also 'fitting in', failure to
Sofia, Bulgaria 106
Solnit, Rebecca 160
Solondz, Todd 59
somatic sensory processing dysfunction 46–7
Somerset House, London 243–4
Sooz 113–14
Sophie Lancaster Foundation, The 54
Soprano, Tony 238
Sparrow, Elizabeth 37–8
speech
  processing 96–7
  see also conversation
spending, compulsive 135–6
spoon theory 107–8, 109–10
sport 46, 60, 61, 64, 68, 79
SSRIs *see* selective serotonin reuptake inhibitors
Star Wars (1977) 48
Starburst magazine 68

Statham, Jason 92
status quo 16, 55, 68–9, 70, 88
Stefania 74
stereotypes, negative 232–3
Steve 97
Steve (ADHDer) 133
stigma 232–3
stimming (self-stimulating behaviour) 57–8
stories *see* other people's stories
stress 32, 33, 47, 118
  childhood 37
  overload 125
  relief 57
  and suicidal ideation *182*, 183
Stuart (author's friend) 130–1
subconscious 46–7, 194
suffering 21
suicidal ideation/thoughts 10, 12, 62, 181–4, *182*, 200–1, 215, 221, 235, 239
suicide 152, 218
  attempted 182
support 239–40
surgical hygiene procedures 31
Sweet and Chicory Tip, The 42

taboos 50, 180
talking things through 41–7, 50
Tamsyn 145
tantrums 178, 179, 223
  see also meltdowns
Tate, Andrew 160
tempers, short 48, 178, 179
Tennant, David 148
tension 47, 56

INDEX

Teresa, Mother 138
testicles, flabby, and male hysteria 9
theory of mind 156–7
therapy 185–97
Third Man, The (1949) 132
Thomas, Adam 66
Thoreau, Henry David 22
thoughts, racing 91–6, 99–101, 112–15, 125–7, 205–6, 208, 216, 243, 248–9
threat perception 40, 74
Thunberg, Greta 159–60
TikTok 10, 73, 205
'time blindness' 123
Times, The (newspaper) 229
Top Hat (1935) 16
Top of the Pops (TV show) 42, 51–2
T'Pau 133
trans people 157–8
  see also LGBT people
transference 190–1
transformation, personal 226–7
trauma 27–34, 36, 221
  and ASD 39
  and executive function 37, 39
  and expectations of the world 40
  long-term impact 52
  and shame 48–9
  and somatic sensory processing dysfunction 46–7
  and the subconscious 46–7
  talking through 41–4, 46–7
  and weirdness 66–7

traumatic brain injury (TBI) 46
Travers, Bill 65
Trent (author's friend) 187–8
tribes, finding 144–6
Trump, Donald 35, 247
trust 191, 192
truth 56
Twitter (X) 201–4

uncertainty 139
unhappiness 7, 15, 21, 40, 217
United Colors of Benetton 156, *156*

'vegan outrage, the' 212
vicious cycles 135
vilification 157–8
visual processing, pre-attentive 46–7
Viz (comic) 98
voice memos 115
Vulcanism 158
vulnerability 51, 168, 234–6
  confident 230–4

Walter, Natasha 50
Warhol, Andy 106
Waters, John 157
wave particle duality 12
Wax, Ruby 229, 240
Webber, Dr 43–4
weirdness 6
  of the human condition 1–2, 23
  realizing that you are odd 53–75

INDEX

Welcome to the Dollhouse (1995) 59–60
Wigtown Book Festival 50
Wilczek, Frank 91–2
Willgoss, Daniel 183
Willgoss, Sue 183
William 120
Williams, Donna 237
Williams, Kenneth 27
Williams, Robin 153
'woke' 247–8
wombs, 'hysterical' 8
women
   'as not funny' 5
   and autism diagnosis 213, 219
   'hysterical' 8–9
   and masking 10
   as peripheral issue 8
   as state of 'weirdness' 5
Woolf, Virginia 139
working memory 37
workplace 16, 54, 103–28
   accommodations 108
   autonomy 115–16
   chopping and changing jobs 120–1
   concealing neurodivergence in 120–1
   and the confidence illusion 117–19
   and creativity 126–7
   and deadlines 105–6, 122
   distracting environment of 104–5, 108, 113–14
   and emails 114–15
   flexible 114
   large corporations 108
   meetings 111–13
   open plan 104–5, 114
   and other people's stories 122–7
   and personal space 104–5
   recruitment procedures 124–5
   and remuneration 115–17
   and timesheets 108
   working around the barriers 110, 111, 114
   working from home 113–14
   working for yourself 108, 110, 136
worry 9
Wyndham, John 64

X (Twitter) 201–4

Y chromosomes 8
Yogi Bear 32
YouGov 136
young carers 214
Young, John Paul 100
Yourgrau, Barry 142

Zen Buddhism 21
Žižek, Slavoj 134–5
Zombi (film series) 247